CHINESE CLASSICS

POPULAR CHINESE HERBAL FORMULAS

A GUIDE FOR THE PRACTITIONER

by Jake Paul Fratkin, OMD, L.Ac.

*Former Chairman, Department of Herbal Medicine
Southwest Acupuncture College
Santa Fe, New Mexico, USA*

SHYA PUBLICATIONS
PO Box 1376
Boulder, Colorado, 80306, USA

COPYRIGHT © 1990 by Jake Paul Fratkin, OMD, L.Ac.
Library of Congress Catalog Card Number: 90-091564
ISBN: O-9626078-1-9

Published and distributed by Shya Publications
PO Box 1376, Boulder, Colorado, 80306, USA
(303) 541-9416

First Printing, July, 1990; Santa Fe, New Mexico
Second Printing, March, 1992; Boulder, Colorado

Library of Congress Catalog in Publication Data
Fratkin, Jake Paul (b. 1948 -)
   Chinese Classics, Popular Chinese Herbal Formulas
   Includes index and glossary
   1. Herbs
   2. Medicine, Chinese

The author wishes to thank Dr. Whitfield Reaves for his encouragement on this project; Mitch Kerman, L.Ac., Efrem Korngold, OMD, L.Ac., Harriet Beinfield, L.Ac. and Z'ev Rosenberg, L.Ac., for their valuable corrections and comments; and my wife, Dominique, for being beautiful.

Type formatting and design: Anne Peacocke
Cover Design: Mary Jonaitis
Cover Photography: Jackie Mathey

Printing: Baker & Johnson, Dexter, Michigan

By the same author:

CHINESE HERBAL PATENT FORMULAS,
Shya Publications, Santa Fe, 1986

THE WQ-10 ELECTRO-ACUPUNCTURE MACHINE,
Paradigm Press, Boston, 1983

This book is intended for practitioners of traditional Chinese medicine who have been trained in Chinese herbal materia medica and prescriptions, as well as traditional diagnosis and differentiation of disease. I have endeavored to make this book useful to practitioners of other healing arts, as well as informed lay persons, but with the caution that difficult cases, or those unresponsive to herbal therapy, be referred to a qualified practitioner of traditional Chinese medicine. I make no claims about the efficacy of these products, only that they are considered useful for many persons when prescribed correctly.

TABLE OF CONTENTS

25. GINSENG & ASTRAGALUS FORMULA

26. GINSENG & ATRACTYLODES FORMULA

27. GINSENG & LONGAN FORMULA

28. GINSENG & TANG KUEI TEN FORMULA

29. GINSENG & ZIZYPHUS FORMULA

30. GINSENG NUTRITIVE FORMULA

31. GUAN JIE FORMULA

32. HOELEN FIVE FORMULA

33. ISATIS FORMULA

34. JADE SCREEN FORMULA

35. JIN GU FORMULA

36. LI DAN FORMULA

37. LONGEVITY FORMULA

38. LYCIUM & REHMANNIA FORMULA

39. MA HUANG & GINKGO PLUS FORMULA

40. MINOR BLUE DRAGON FORMULA

41. MINOR BUPLEURUM FORMULA

42. OPHIOPOGON & ASARUM FORMULA

43. OPHIOPOGON PLUS FORMULA

44. PASSWAN FORMULA

45. PINELLIA & MAGNOLIA FORMULA

46. PINELLIA "X" FORMULA

47. PLATYCODON & FRITILLARIA FORMULA

48. PUERARIA FORMULA

49. PUERARIA "N" FORMULA

50. REHMANNIA EIGHT PLUS FORMULA

51. REHMANNIA SIX FORMULA

CHINESE CLASSICS, POPULAR CHINESE HERBAL FORMULAS

INTRODUCTION

This short work is intended as a practitioner's guide to a group of Chinese herbal products readily available in the United States. The complete line of products described here is offered by McZand Herbal, Inc. in the form of herbal liquid extracts. Many of the products are also offered by Sun Ten Corporation, and distributed by Brion Corporation, as granular extracts, as well as the companies Qualiherb, Mintang Formulas, and Kanpo Formulas. Several of the products are prepared in pill form as Chinese patent medicines.

These herbal products have been chosen for their known effectiveness for a variety of complaints. Many are based on classical prescriptions dating back to the Shang Han Lun, circa 200 AD, while others have been in use for the last 300 years. Their clinical usefulness is well known and appreciated in China and Japan, as well as in this country.

As herbal liquid extracts, the products are normally dosed at two to three droppers, two to three times per day. Although the manufacturer feels that the extract can be taken directly into the mouth, I recommend that the liquid be put into a cup, with a small amount of boiling water added, and steeped for five minutes. This will dispel the alcohol, and minimize heating reactions in sensitive patients. If there is no sensitivity, room temperature water is adequate. The manufacturer, McZand Herbal, Inc., feels that the quality of their extraction process allows for maximum medicinal effect, with a cost savings for the patient. The advantage of liquid drops also is high patient compliance.

Granule extracts as offered by Sun Ten Formulas (Brion Corp.), Qualiherb, Mintang Formulas, and Kanpo Formulas, are taken with their enclosed white spoon; normal dosing is one to two spoonfuls, two to three times per day.

Doses for the Chinese herbal patent medicines are taken according to the recommendation on the box. Doses are also clearly indicated in my book, **Chinese Herbal Patent Formulas**.

I believe that these herbal products can provide low cost, high quality health care for many patients. The herbal products described here accelerate the body's ability to heal itself, and can be significantly effective over a correct period of time.

These products are best administered by a trained practitioner of oriental medicine, one who has studied well the individual herbs and prescriptions. Other doctors, as well as informed consumers, can use this book for treating common health complaints by using the indications set forth with each product, as well as the index.

These products are basically safe. Negative effects to any Chinese herbal product may include nausea, headache, and irritability. If the prescription chosen is correct, and these effects occur, it is probably that the patient is being overdosed. Reducing the quantity or frequency will usually alleviate the problem. Some patients, about five percent of the population, cannot tolerate herbs in any dose; these people are usually supersensitive to all forms of medication, as well as acupuncture. Here, heeding their warnings of sensitivity before prescribing may be in order.

1. ANEM–PHELLO & REHMANNIA FORMULA

Deficiency heat

Zhi Bai Di Huang Wan
"Anemarrhena, Phellodendron, Rehmannia Decoction"

Energetic and functional presentation:

Deficiency of *yin* with heat or fire
Deficiency of kidney *yin*
Blood heat due to deficiency of *yin*
Deficiency of liver *yin*
Deficiency of stomach *yin*

Tongue: Dry coat; glossy red, or red at sides
Pulse: Thin, rapid

Symptoms and applications:

Dry throat and mouth
Hot flashing
Hot palms and soles
Insomnia
Low grade fevers

Night sweats
Premature ejaculations
Restlessness
Spermatorrhea
Tidal fevers

Herbal prescription:

Rehmannia *Shu Di*	TBI*	Dioscorea *Shan Yao*	TQi
Anemarrhena *Zhi Mu*	CIH	Poria *Fu Ling*	DD
Phellodendron *Huang Bai*	CDH	Alisma *Ze Xie*	DD
Cornus *Shan Zhu Ru*	AH	Moutan *Mu Dan Pi*	CBH

Availability:

1. Zand Chinese Classics, McZand Herbal, Inc; herbal liquid extract.
2. As **Anemarrhena, Phellodendron and Rehmannia Formula**; extract granules. **
3. As **Eight Flavor Tea**; Chinese patent medicine; pills.
4. As **Temper Fire**; Jade Pharmacy; herbal liquid extract or tablets.

* For herbal codes, see **Herbal Naming Cross Reference**, p. 72.
** From Brion-Sunten, Qualiherb, Mintang Formulas and Kanpo Formulas. See Suppliers of Products, p. 105.

2. ASTRAGALUS & GANODERMA FORMULA

Immune deficiency due to deficient qi and yin

Huang Qi Ling Zhi San
"Astragalus, Ganoderma Powder"

Energetic and functional presentation:

Deficiency of spleen *qi*
Deficiency of *wei qi*
Deficiency of lung *qi*
Deficiency of lung *yin*
Deficiency of heart *qi*
Deficiency of heart *yin*

Tongue: Thin; may be reddish, may be pale
Pulse: Thin, weak, may be slightly rapid

Symptoms and applications:

ARC (AIDS Related Complex)
Chronic Fatigue Syndrome
Dry cough
Post-fever fatigue
Post-partum fatigue
Post-surgical fatigue
Tuberculosis
Chronic myocarditis
Weak heart in the aged

Herbal prescription:

Astragalus *Huang Qi*	TQi	Dendrobrium *Shi Hu*	TYi
Ganoderma *Ling Zhi*	TQi	Schizandra *Wu Wei Zi*	AH
Ligustrum *Nu Zhen Zi*	TYi	Lycium Gou *Qi Zi*	TBI
Codonopsis *Dang Shen*	TQi	Polygonum *He Shou Wu*	TBI
Eleutheroginseng *Ci Wu Jia*	TQi	Angelica *Dang Gui*	TBI
Quinquefolium *Xi Yang Shen*	TYi	Eucommia *Du Zhong*	TYa
Atractylodes *Bai Zhu*	TQi	Citrus *Chen Pi*	RSQ
Ophiopogon *Mai Men Dong*	TYi	Glycerrhiza *Gan Cao*	TQi

Comments:

1. In viral problems, including AIDS, myocarditis, and Chronic Fatigue Syndrome, consider combining with **Isatis Formula**.
2. This formula should be taken over a period of months, as long as dry symptoms persist.

Availability:

1. Zand Chinese Classics, McZand Herbal, Inc; herbal liquid extract.

3. BUPLEURUM & CINNAMON FORMULA

Digestive disturbance

Chai Hu Gui Zhi Tang

"Bupleurum, Cinnamomum Decoction"

Energetic and functional presentation:

Dysharmony of liver and spleen–stomach
Stagnation of liver and gallbladder*qi*
Stagnation of stomach *qi*
Wind-cold invasion with pre-existing deficiency
Stomach phlegm
Deficiency of spleen *qi*
Liver heat

Tongue: Pale, swollen; moderate to greasy yellow or white coat
Pulse: Weak wiry; may be slippery;
wiry in liver position, weak in spleen position.

Symptoms and applications:

Abdominal distention	Gallbladder congestion
Abdominal pain	Headache
Common cold with	Irritability
chest constriction	Muscular tension
Epigastric pain	Nausea
Fat digestion poor	Vertebral subluxation
Flatulence	Vomiting

Herbal prescription:

Bupleurum *Chai Hu*	DWH	Jujube *Da Zao*		TQi
Pinellia *Ban Xia*	TPD	Scutellaria *Huang Qin*		CDH
Cinnamomum *Gui Zhi*	DWC	Glycerrhiza *Gan Cao*		TQi
Paeonia *Bai Shao*	TBl	Zingiberis *Sheng Jiang*		DWC
Codonopsis *Dang Shen*	TQi			

Comments:

1. Bupleurum formulas may open and invigorate the liver too quickly, causing side effects of symptom aggravation, digestive problems, or irritability. If this is the case, reduce dosage.

Availability:

1. Zand Chinese Classics, McZand Herbal, Inc; herbal liquid extract.
2. As **Bupleurum and Cinnamon Combination**; extract granules.

4. BUPLEURUM & DRAGON BONE FORMULA

Irritability; Drug and smoking withdrawal

Chai Hu Jia Long Gu Mu Li Tang
"Bupleurum with Draconis, Ostrea Decoction"

Energetic and functional presentation:

Stagnation of liver *qi*
Rising liver *yang*
Disturbed *shen*
Deficiency of spleen *qi*
Stomach phlegm
Large Intestine heat
Liver heat

Tongue: Red sides; occasional moderate to greasy yellow or white coat
Pulse: Wiry; especially in liver or gallbladder position; slightly rapid

Symptoms and applications:

Epilepsy
Headache
Hypertension
Insomnia
Irritability

Mania
Palpitation
Restlessness
Smoking or drug withdrawal

Herbal prescription:

Bupleurum *Chai Hu*	DWH	Draconis *Long Gu*		CS
Pinellia *Ban Xia*	TPD	Ostrea *Mu Li*		CS
Cinnamomum *Gui Zhi*	DWC	Zingiberis *Sheng Jiang*		WI
Poria *Fu Ling*	DD	Jujube *Da Zao*		TQi
Scutellaria *Huang Qin*	CDH	Rheum *Da Huang*		Pu
Codonopsis *Dang Shen*	TQi			

Comments:

1. This formula may cause loose stools. If this occurs, reduce dosage.
2. Bupleurum formulas may open and invigorate the liver too quickly, causing side effects of symptom aggravation, digestive problems, or irritability. If this is the case, reduce dosage.

Availability:

1. Zand Chinese Classics, McZand Herbal, Inc; herbal liquid extract.
2. As **Bupleurum and Dragon Bone Combination**; extract granules.
3. As **Ease Plus**; Health Concerns; tablets.

5. BUPLEURUM & PEONY FORMULA

Premenstrual syndrome with liver heat

Dan Zhi Xiao Yao San
"Moutan, Gardenia Free (and) Relaxed Powder"

Energetic and functional presentation:

Stagnation of liver *qi* and blood
Liver heat
Deficiency of liver blood
Dysharmony of liver and spleen
Deficiency of spleen *qi*

Tongue: Red sides, occasionally pale body
Pulse: Wiry, especially in the liver position; slightly rapid, thin

Symptoms and applications:

Abdominal distension	Irregular menstruation
Breast distension	Irritability
Dizziness	Poor appetite
Food allergies	Premenstrual syndrome (PMS)
Headache	Red eye
Hot flashing (menopause)	Restlessness
Infertility	

Herbal prescription:

Bupleurum *Chai Hu*	DWH	Zingiberis *Sheng Jiang*	DWC
Paeonia *Bai Shao*	TBI	Moutan *Mu Dan Pi*	CBH
Angelica *Dang Gui*	TBI	Gardenia *Zhi Zi*	CIH
Poria *Fu Ling*	DD	Glycerrhiza *Gan Cao*	TQi
Atractylodes *Bai Zhu*	TQi	Mentha *Bo He*	DWH

Comments:

1. This formula is primarily used for menstrual disorders, where heat in the liver is evident.
2. Bupleurum formulas may open and invigorate the liver too quickly, causing side effects of symptom aggravation, digestive problems, or irritability. If this is the case, reduce dosage.
3. This formula is best administered between ovulation and onset of the period.
4. May be useful as a preventative of adverse menopausal symptoms, taken for one or two years prior.

Availability:

1. Zand Chinese Classics, McZand Herbal, Inc; herbal liquid extract.
2. As **Bupleurum and Peony Combination**; extract granules.
3. As **Relaxed Wanderer**; Jade Pharmacy; herbal liquid extract or tablets.

6. BUPLEURUM & TANG KUEI FORMULA

Premenstrual syndrome

Xiao Yao San
"Free and Relaxed Powder"

Energetic and functional presentation:

Stagnation of liver *qi* and blood
Deficiency of liver blood
Deficiency of spleen *qi*
Dysharmony of liver and spleen

Tongue: Occasionally pale body; slight red to sides
Pulse: Wiry, especially in the liver position; slightly rapid, thin

Symptoms and applications:

Abdominal distension	Infertility
Blurry vision	Irregular menstruation
Breast distension	Irritability
Depression	Poor appetite
Dizziness	Premenstrual syndrome (PMS)
Food allergies	Premenstrual constipation
Headache	Tension

Herbal prescription:

Bupleurum *Chai Hu*	DWH	Atractylodes *Bai Zhu*	TQi
Paeonia *Bai Shao*	TBI	Zingiberis *Sheng Jiang*	DWC
Angelica *Dang Gui*	TBI	Glycerrhiza *Gan Cao*	TQi
Poria *Fu Ling*	DD	Mentha *Bo He*	DWH

Comments:

1. This formula is primarily used for menstrual and premenstrual disorders, where heat is not evident.
2. Bupleurum formulas may open and invigorate the liver too quickly, causing side effects of symptom aggravation, digestive problems, or irritability. If this is the case, reduce dosage.
3. This formula is best administered between ovulation and onset of the period.

Availability:

1. Zand Chinese Classics, McZand Herbal, Inc; herbal liquid extract.
2. As **Bupleurum and Tang–kuei Combination**; extract granules.
3. As **Hsiao Yao Wan**, Chinese patent medicine; pills.

7. BU TIAO FORMULA

Blood stagnation in the uterus due to cold

Bu Xue Tiao Jing Tang
"Nourish Blood, Adjust Period Decoction"

Energetic and functional presentation:

Cold in the uterus
Blood stagnation in the uterus
Deficiency of kidney *qi* and *yang*
Deficiency of *qi* and blood
Bleeding due to *qi* deficiency

Tongue: Pale, dark
Pulse: Choppy, weak, thin

Symptoms and applications:

Amenorrhea	Infertility
Dysmenorrhea	Irregular periods
Fatigue	Uterine bleeding

Herbal prescription:

Cyperus *Xiang Fu*	RSQ	Artemesia *Ai Ye*	SB
Rosa *Jin Ying Zi*	AH	Capsella *Ji Cai*	CBH
Millettia *Ji Xue Teng*	IB	Codonopsis *Dang Shen*	TQi
Litsea *Dou Chi Jing*	WI	Atractylodes *Cang Zhu*	TSD
Loranthus *Sang Ji Sheng*	TYi	Glycerrhiza *Gan Cao*	TQi
Leonurus *Yi Mu Cao*	IB	Gelatinum *E Jiao*	TBI
Alpinia Gao *Liang Jiang*	WI	Cinnamomum *Rou Gui*	WI

Availability:

1. Zand Chinese Classics, McZand Herbal, Inc; herbal liquid extract.
2. As **Butiao Tablets**; Chinese patent medicine; tablets.

8. CAPILLARIS & HOELEN FORMULA

Edema

Yin Chen Wu Ling Tang

"Artemesia, Five Poria Decoction"

Energetic and functional presentation:

Accumulation of damp and water

Tongue: Swollen, red sides, wet; possibly a yellow coat
Pulse: Wide, soft; possibly rapid; occasionally slippery

Symptoms and applications:

Ascites	Jaundice
Ascites due to jaundice	Lower back pain
or cirrhosis	Painful urination
Diarrhea	Scrotal hydrocele
Edema	Headache due to viral
Hematuria	encephalia

Herbal prescription:

Artemesia *Yin Chen Hao*	DD	Atractylodes *Cang Zhu*	TSD
Poria *Fu Ling*	DD	Alisma *Ze Xie*	DD
Polyporous *Zhu Ling*	DD	Cinnamomum *Gui Zhi*	DWC

Availability:

1. Zand Chinese Classics, McZand Herbal, Inc; herbal liquid extract.
2. As extract granules.

9. CARDAMON & FENNEL FORMULA

Epigastric pain

An Zhong Tang
"Peaceful Center"

Energetic and functional presentation:

Hyperacidity of the stomach
Stagnation of blood in the stomach
Stagnation of stomach *qi* with cold

Tongue: Dark
Pulse: Choppy or wiry

Symptoms and applications:

Epigastric distension
Epigastric pain
Ulcer
Vomiting of blood

Herbal prescription:

Cinnamomum *Gui Zhi*	DWC	Amomum *Sha Ren*	TSD
Corydalis *Yan Hu Suo*	IB	Glycerrhiza *Gan Cao*	TQi
Ostrea *Mu Li*	CS	Alpinia *Gao Liang Jiang*	WI
Foeniculum *Hui Xiang*	WI		

Availability:

1. Zand Chinese Classics, McZand Herbal, Inc; herbal liquid extract.
2. As extract granules.

10. CARTHAMUS & PERSICA FORMULA

Menstrual cramps

Hong Hua Tao Ren Tang

"Carthamus, Persica Decoction"

Energetic and functional presentation:

Stagnation of liver blood
Stagnation of uterus blood
Stagnation of liver *qi*

Tongue: Dark, or with purple spots
Pulse: Choppy or wiry, hesitant

Symptoms and applications:

Amenorrhea
Dysmenorrhea
Irregular menstruation
Ovarian cyst

Swollen liver
  (hepatomegaly)
Traumatic injury
Uterine fibroids

Herbal prescription:

Rehmannia *Sheng Di*	CBH	Corydalis *Yan Hu Suo*	IB
Carthamus *Hong Hua*	IB	Angelica *Dang Gui*	TBI
Persica *Tao Ren*	IB	Ligusticum *Chuan Xiong*	IB
Salvia *Dan Shen*	IB	Cyperus *Xiang Fu*	RSQ
Paeonia *Chi Shao*	IB	Citrus *Qing Pi*	RSQ

Comments:

1. This formula is primarily used for dysmenorrhea (menstrual cramps), and hepatomegaly.
2. Contraindicated during pregnancy.

Availability:

1. Zand Chinese Classics, McZand Herbal, Inc; herbal liquid extract.

11. CHIANGHUO & TURMERIC FORMULA

Painful arthralgia of upper limbs

Chuan Bi Tang

"Relieve Bi Syndrome Decoction"

Energetic and functional presentation:

Wind–cold-damp obstruction in the channels
Blood stagnation in the channels

Tongue: Possibly wet; possibly dark
Pulse: Superficial; wiry or choppy

Symptoms and applications:

Arthritis
Bursitis of shoulder or hip
Difficulty moving joints and limbs

Rheumatism, especially upper limbs
Spasms
Wind–damp Bi syndrome

Herbal prescription:

Astragalus Huang Qi	TQi	Siler Fang Feng	DWC
Notopterygium Qiang Huo	DWC	Zingiberis Sheng Jiang	DWC
Curcuma Jiang Huang	IB	Jujube Da Zao	TQi
Angelica Dang Gui	TBI	Glycerrhiza Gan Cao	TQi
Paeonia Chi Shao	IB		

Comments:

1. This formula is preferred in wind-cold-damp Bi syndrome where pain is the predominant symptom.

Availability:

1. Zand Chinese Classics, McZand Herbal, Inc; herbal liquid extract.
2. As **Chianghuo and Turmeric Combination**; extract granules.

12. CHUAN XIONG FORMULA
Wind-cold with headache
Chuan Xiong Cha Tiao Tang
"Ligusticum (with) Green Tea Mix Decotion"

Energetic and functional presentation:

Wind-cold invasion into channels
Stagnation of *qi* and blood in channels

Tongue: Normal; may be pale or dark
Pulse: Superficial, excessive, wiry

Symptoms and applications:

Aching neck and shoulders	Headache
Common cold without fever	Sinus headache

Herbal prescription:

Mentha *Bo He*	DWH	Notopterygium *Qiang Huo*	DWC
Ligusticum *Chuan Xiong*	IB	Siler *Fang Feng*	DWC
Schizonepeta *Jing Jie*	DWC	Glycerrhiza *Gan Cao*	TQi
Angelica *Bai Zhi*	DWC	Asarum *Xi Xln*	DWC

Comments:

1. Primarily for wind-cold headache.
2. The original classical formula recommended taking with strong tea to enhance wind-dispersing effect.

Availability:

1. Zand Chinese Classics, McZand Herbal, Inc; herbal liquid extract.
2. As **Cnidium and Tea Formula**; extract granules.
3. As **Chuan Qiong Cha Tiao Wan**; Chinese patent medicine; pills.

13. CINNAMON & HOELEN FORMULA

Blood stagnation in the uterus

Gui Zhi Fu Ling Tang
"Cinnamomum, Poria Decoction"

Energetic and functional presentation:

Blood stagnation in the uterus
Cold uterus

Tongue: Dark; or with purple spots
Pulse: Choppy or wiry

Symptoms and applications:

Abdominal pain	Irregular menstruation
Amenorrhea	Leukorrhea
Dysmenorrhea	Retained placenta
Endometriosis	Uterine fibroids
Infertility	

Herbal prescription:

Cinnamomum *Gui Zhi*	DWC	Persica *Tao Ren*	IB
Poria *Fu Ling*	DD	Moutan *Mu Dan Pi*	CBH
Paeonia *Chi Shao*	IB		

Availability:

1. Zand Chinese Classics, McZand Herbal, Inc; herbal liquid extract.
2. As extract granules.

14. CITRUS & CRATAEGUS FORMULA

Food stagnation

Bao He Tang

"Protect (the) Harmonious Decoction"

Energetic and functional presentation:

Stagnation of food
Accumulation of phlegm and phlegm–heat in stomach
Stagnation of stomach *qi*
Stagnation of heat blood

Tongue: Thick yellow greasy coat
Pulse: Slippery

Symptoms and applications:

Abdominal distension
Belching
Epigastric distension
Epigastric pain
Erratic stools (pasty, constipation, diarrhea)
Flatulence
Food stagnation
Hangover
High blood cholesterol
Hypertension

Herbal prescription:

Crataegus *Shan Zha*	RFS	Forsythia *Lian Qiao*	CTH
Pinellia *Ban Xia*	TPD	Massa Fermentata *Shen Chu*	RFS
Poria *Fu Ling*	DD	Raphanus *Lai Fu Zi*	RFS
Citrus *Chen Pi*	RSQ		

Comments:

1. This formula has been shown to reduce blood cholesterol.

Availability:

1. Zand Chinese Classics, McZand Herbal, Inc; herbal liquid extract.
2. As **Citrus and Crataegus Combination**; extract granules.

15. CITRUS & PINELLIA FORMULA
Phlegm

Er Chen Tang
"Two-Aged Decoction"

Energetic and functional presentation:

Stomach phlegm–damp
Lung phlegm-damp

Tongue: Pale, swollen; white greasy coat
Pulse: Weak, or slippery; may be excessive
in stomach or lung position

Symptoms and applications:

Chronic cough with phlegm
Diarrhea or loose stools
Dizziness
Epigastric distension
Goiter
Hangover

Lung phlegm–damp, chronic
Nausea
Poor appetite
Vomiting
Watery phlegm in mouth

Herbal prescription:

Pinellia *Ban Xia*   TPD
Citrus *Chen Pi*   RSQ
Poria *Fu Ling*   DD

Glycerrhiza *Gan Cao*   TQi
Zingiberis *Sheng Jiang*   DWS

Availability:

1. Zand Chinese Classics, McZand Herbal, Inc; herbal liquid extract.
2. As **Citrus and Pinellia Combination**; extract granules.
3. As **Erh Chen Wan**; Chinese patent medicine; pills.

16. CLEMATIS & STEPHANIA FORMULA

Painful lower limbs and joints

Shu Jing Huo Xue Tang

"Disperse Channels Invigorate Blood Decoction"

Energetic and functional presentation:

Stagnation of wind–cold–damp in the channels
Stagnation of *qi* and blood in the channels

Tongue: Swollen
Pulse: Superficial, choppy

Symptoms and applications:

Arthralgia	Edema in the limbs
Arthritis	Low back pain
Bi syndrome,	Painful joints and limbs (lower)
wind–cold–damp type	Rheumatism
Difficult movement	Sciatica

Herbal prescription:

Paeonia *Chi Shao*	IB	Notopterygium *Qiang Huo*	DWC
Rehmannia *Shu Di*	TBI	Citrus *Chen Pi*	RSQ
Persica *Tao Ren*	IB	Siler *Fang Feng*	DWC
Angelica *Dang Gui*	TBI	Gentiana *Long Dan Cao*	CDH
Ligusticum *Chuan Xiong*	IB	Achyranthes *Huai Niu Xi*	TYi
Atractylodes *Cang Zhu*	TSD	Angelica *Bai Zhi*	DWC
Poria *Fu Ling*	DD	Zingiberis *Sheng Jiang*	DWC
Clematis *Wei Ling Xian*	DWD	Glycerrhiza *Gan Cao*	TQi
Stephania *Fang Ji*	DD		

Availability:

1. Zand Chinese Classics, McZand Herbal, Inc; herbal liquid extract.
2. As **Clematis and Stephania Combination**; extract granules.
3. As **Mobility 2**; Health Concerns; tablets.

17. COIX FORMULA

Painful upper limbs with damp accumulation

Yi Yi Ren Tang
"Coix Decoction"

Energetic and functional presentation:

Wind–cold–damp in channels

Tongue: Occasionally wet or swollen
Pulse: Superficial; tight, choppy or slippery

Symptoms and applications:

Arthralgia	Difficult movement
Arthritis	Edema in the limbs
Bi syndrome,	Painful joints and limbs (upper)
wind–cold–damp type	Rheumatism

Herbal prescription:

Coix *Yi Yi Ren*	DD	Paeonia *Bai Shao*	TBI
Ephedra *Ma Huang*	DWC	Cinnamomum *Gui Zhi*	DWC
Atractylodes *Bai Zhu*	TQi	Glycerrhiza *Gan Cao*	TQi
Angelica *Dang Gui*	TBI		

Comments:

1. This formula is preferred in wind-cold-damp *Bi* syndrome where damp is the predominant symptom.

Availability:

1. Zand Chinese Classics, McZand Herbal, Inc; herbal liquid extract.
2. As **Coix Combination**; extract granules.
3. As **Mobility I**, Health Concerns.

18. COPTIS & SCUTE FORMULA

Liver heat, blood heat; Bacterial infections

Huang Lian Jie Du Tang
"Coptis Dispel Toxin Decoction"

Energetic and functional presentation:

Toxic heat
Liver heat
Blood heat

Tongue: Bright red
Pulse: Excessive, bounding, wiry, rapid

Symptoms and applications:

Bacterial infections
Bleeding: nose, gums,
    urine, stools, or uterus
Boils and carbuncles
Fever with constipation
Fever with delerium

High fever
Hives
Rheumatic fever
Strept throat
Styes

Herbal prescription:

Scutellaria *Huang Qin*	CDH	Gardenia *Zhi Zi*	CIH
Phellodendron *Huang Bai*	CDH	Coptis *Huang Lian*	CDH

Comments:

1. Use until fever or heat condition is reduced. Discontinue or lower dosage in the event of diarrhea. Prolonged use will injure the spleen-pancreas and stomach.
2. In heat conditions, it may be important to add boiling water to herbal extracts, to neutralize the heating effects of alcohol.

Availability:

1. Zand Chinese Classics, McZand Herbal, Inc; herbal liquid extract.
2. As **Coptis and Scute Combination**; extract granules.

19. CURING FORMULA
Digestive complaints
Kang Ning Wan
"Healthy Quiet Pills"

Energetic and functional presentation:

Stagnation of phlegm in stomach
Stagnation of stomach *qi*
Accumulation of spleen damp
Toxic wind–heat invasion into stomach
Deficiency of spleen *qi*

Tongue: Occasionally swollen; greasy white or yellow coat
Pulse: Occasionally slippery; weak in spleen position;
occasionally excess in stomach position

Symptoms and applications:

Abdominal distension
Abdominal pain
Epigastric distension
Epigastric pain
Erratic stools (diarrhea, loose,
pasty, or constipation)
Flatulence

Food poisoning
Food stagnation
Hangover
Morning sickness
Motion sickness
Nausea
Stomach flu

Herbal prescription:

Poria *Fu Ling*	DD	Trichosanthes *Tian Hua Fen*	TPH
Coix *Yi Yi Ren*	DD	Oryza *Gu Ya*	RFS
Magnolia *Hou Po*	TSD	Massa Fermentata *Shen Chu*	RFS
Atractylodes *Bai Zhu*	TQi	Gastrodia *Tian Ma*	SL
Pogostemon *Huo Xiang*	TSD	Chrysanthemum *Ju Hua*	DWH
Pueraria *Ge Gen*	DWH	Citrus *Chen Pi*	RSQ
Angelica *Bai Zhi*	DWC	Mentha *Bo He*	DWH
Saussurea *Mu Xiang*	RSQ		

Availability:

1. Zand Chinese Classics, McZand Herbal, Inc; herbal liquid extract.
2. As **Pill Curing**; Chinese patent medicine; pills.

20. DIANTHUS FORMULA
Urinary tract infections

Ba Zheng Tang

"Eight–Righteous Decoction"

Energetic and functional presentation:

Damp–heat in bladder
Damp–heat in kidney

Tongue: Red, or red on sides; yellow coat in back
Pulse: Rapid; forceful in proximal (kidney) positions

Symptoms and applications:

Bladder stone	Pelvic inflammatory disease
Kidney infection	Prostatitis
Painful or difficult urination	Urinary tract infection

Herbal prescription:

Talcum *Hua Shi*	DD	Plantago *Che Qian Zi*	DD
Dianthus *Qu Mai*	DD	Juncus *Deng Xin Cao*	DD
Akebia *Mu Tong*	DD	Rheum *Da Huang*	Pu
Polygonum *Bian Xu*	DD	Glycerrhiza *Gan Cao*	TQi
Gardenia *Zhi Zi*	CIH		

Comments:

1. Contraindicated during pregnancy.

Availability:

1. Zand Chinese Classics, McZand Herbal, Inc; herbal liquid extract.
2. As extract granules.

21. DU HUO & LORANTHUS FORMULA

Weak back and legs due to cold

Du Huo Ji Sheng Tang
"Angelica *Du Huo*, Loranthus Decoction"

Energetic and functional presentation:

Stagnation and cold in the channels
Deficiency of kidney *yang*
Wind–cold–damp in the channels
Deficiency of liver blood

Tongue: May be pale, or dark
Pulse: Weak in the kidney positions

Symptoms and applications:

Arthralgia	Stiff joints
Bi syndrome	Stiffness in walking
Lower back pain	Cold back and knees

Herbal prescription:

Angelica *Du Huo*	DWD	Asarum *Xi Xin*	DWC
Loranthus *Sang Ji Sheng*	TYI	Ginseng *Ren Shen*	TQi
Poria *Fu Ling*	DD	Cinnamomum *Rou Gui*	WI
Rehmannia *Shu Di Huang*	TBI	Angelica *Dang Gui*	TBI
Eucommia *Du Zhong*	TYa	Paeonia *Bai Shao*	TBI
Gentiana *Qin Jiao*	DWD	Ligusticum *Chuan Xiong*	IB
Achyranthes *Niu Xi*	TYi	Glycerrhiza *Gan Cao*	TQi
Siler *Fang Feng*	DWC		

Comments:

1. This is the formula of choice for weak lower back due to kidney *yang* deficiency.
2. Caution during pregnancy.

Availability:

1. Zand Chinese Classics, McZand Herbal, Inc; herbal liquid extract.
2. As **Tu-huo and Vaeicum Combination**; extract granules.
3. As **Du Huo Jisheng Wan**; Chinese patent medicine; pills.

22. FOUR GENTLEMEN FORMULA

Deficiency of spleen qi

Si Jun Zi Tang
"Four Sage Decoction"

Energetic and functional presentation:

Deficiency of spleen *qi*

Tongue: Pale, slightly swollen
Pulse: Weak, especially in the spleen position

Symptoms and applications:

Fatigue
Poor digestion
Poor appetite
Flatulence
Pasty Stools

Herbal prescription:

Codonopsis *Dang Shen*	TQi	Poria *Fu Ling*	DD
Atractylodes *Bai Zhu*	TQi	Glycerrhiza *Gan Cao*	TQi

Comments:

1. This is the foundation formula for deficiency of spleen *qi*.

Availability:

1. Zand Chinese Classics, McZand Herbal, Inc; herbal liquid extract.
2. As **Four Major Herbs Combination**; extract granules.

23. GASTRODIA & UNCARIA FORMULA

Hypertension; Headache

Tian Ma Gou Teng Yin

"Gastrodia, Uncaria Cool Decoction"

Energetic and functional presentation:

Liver wind
Rising liver yang
Deficiency of liver yin
Liver heat

Tongue: Red on sides
Pulse: Superficial, thin, slightly rapid; excess in gallbladder position, thin in liver position

Symptoms and applications:

Dizziness	Hypertension
Dry eyes	Light–headed
Ear–ringing	Pressure behind eyes
Headache	

Herbal prescription:

Gastrodia Tian Ma	SL	Leonurus Yi Mu Cao	IB
Uncaria Gou Teng	SL	Polygonum Ye Jiao Teng	CS
Loranthus Sang Ji Sheng	TYi	Poria Fu Ling	DD
Eucommia Du Zhong	TYa	Haliotis Shi Jue Ming	SL
Cyathula Chuan Niu Xi	IB	Gardenia Zhi Zi	CIH
Scutellaria Huang Qin	CDH		

Availability:

1. Zand Chinese Classics, McZand Herbal, Inc; herbal liquid extract.
2. As **Gastrodia and Uncaria Combination**; extract granules.

24. GENTIANA FORMULA
Urinary tract infection; Herpes; Red eye
Long Dan Xie Gan Tang
"Gentiana Purge Liver Decoction"

Energetic and functional presentation:

Bladder damp–heat
Liver–gallbladder damp–heat
Liver–gallbladder fire

Tongue: Red sides, yellow greasy coat
Pulse: Wiry, rapid, occasionally thin;
excessive in gallbladder or liver positions

Symptoms and applications:

Bitter taste in mouth
Boils along gallbladder
channel
Eye pressure
Gallstones
Headache
Hepatitis
Herpes (oral or genital)
Leukorrhea

Pelvic inflammatory disease
Prostatitis
Red eye
Scrotal eczema
Testicles swollen
Urinary tract infection
Urine concentrated or painful
Vaginitis

Herbal prescription:

Scutellaria *Huang Qin*	CDH		Plantago *Che Qian Zi*	DD
Rehmannia *Sheng Di*	CBH		Alisma *Ze Xie*	DD
Gentiana *Long Dan Cao*	CDH		Gardenia *Zhi Zi*	CIH
Angelica *Dang Gui Wei*	TBI		Akebia *Mu Tong*	DD
Bupleurum *Chai Hu*	DWH		Glycerrhiza *Gan Cao*	TQi

Comments:

1. In heat conditions, it may be important to add boiling water to neutralize the effects of alcohol.

Availability:

1. Zand Chinese Classics, McZand Herbal, Inc; herbal liquid extract.
2. As **Gentiana Combination**; extract granules.
3. As **Lung Tan Xie Gan Wan**; Chinese patent medicine; pills.
4. As **Quell Fire**; Jade Pharmacy, K'an Herb Company; herbal liquid extract or tablets.

25. GINSENG & ASTRAGALUS FORMULA

Deficiency of spleen qi

Bu Zhong Yi Qi Tang
"Tonify the Center, Invigorate *Qi* Decoction"

Energetic and functional presentation:

Deficiency of spleen *qi*
Sinking of spleen *qi* and *yang*
Dysharmony of spleen, stomach, liver, and gallbladder

Tongue: Slightly swollen; occasionally pale
Pulse: Weak, especially in the spleen position

Symptoms and applications:

Abdominal distension
Deficiency uterine bleeding
Diarrhea
Fatigue
Flatulence
Hernia

Hypoglycemia
Loose or erratic stools
Prostatitis, chronic
Poor digestion
Prolapse of intestine, rectum,
  or uterus

Herbal prescription:

Astragalus *Huang Qi*	TQi	Cimicifuga *Sheng Ma*	DWH
Atractylodes *Bai Zhu*	TQi	Jujube *Da Zao*	TQi
Codonopsis *Dang Shen*	TQi	Zingiberis *Sheng Jiang*	DWC
Angelica *Dang Gui*	TBI	Glycerrhiza *Gan Cao*	TQi
Bupleurum *Chai Hu*	DWH	Ginseng *Ren Shen*	TQi
Citrus *Chen Pi*	RSQ		

Availability:

1. Zand Chinese Classics, McZand Herbal, Inc; herbal liquid extract.
2. As **Ginseng and Astragalus Combination**; extract granules.
3. As **Central Chi Pills**; Chinese patent medicine; pills.
4. As **Arouse Vigor**; Jade Pharmacy, K'an Herb Company; herbal liquid extract or tablets.

26. GINSENG & ATRACTYLODES FORMULA

Loose stools due to spleen deficiency

Shen Ling Bai Zhu Tang

"Ginseng, Poria, Atractylodes Decoction"

Energetic and functional presentation:

Deficiency of spleen *qi*
Accumulation of spleen damp

Tongue: Swollen, may be pale; wet;
occasionally white greasy coat
Pulse: Soft or slippery, especially in spleen position

Symptoms and applications:

Abdominal distension	Leukorrhea
Diarrhea	Loose stools
Edema	Morning sickness
Fatigue	Nausea
Gas or flatulence	Poor appetite
Indigestion	Weak muscle strength

Herbal prescription:

Coix *Yi Yi Ren*	DD	Ginseng *Ren Shen*	TQi
Dolichoris *Bai Bian Dou*	CSH	Atractylodes *Bai Zhu*	TQi
Nelumbo *Lian Zi*	AH	Platycodon *Jie Geng*	TPD
Dioscorea *Shan Yao*	TQi	Amomum *Sha Ren*	TSD
Poria *Fu Ling*	DD	Glycerrhiza *Zhi Gan Cao*	TQi

Comments:

1. This is the formula of choice for loose stools due to spleen *qi* deficiency.

Availability:

1. Zand Chinese Classics, McZand Herbal, Inc; herbal liquid extract.
2. As extract granules.
3. As **Shen Ling Baizhu Pian**; Chinese patent medicine; pills.

27. GINSENG & LONGAN FORMULA

Insomnia, Palpitations

Gui Pi Tang
"Restore Spleen Decoction"

Energetic and functional presentation:

Tonify spleen *qi*
Nourish heart blood
Calm *shen*

Tongue: Pale
Pulse: Weak, thin;
weak in spleen and heart positions

Symptoms and applications:

Anemia
Anxiety or nervousness
Deficiency uterine bleeding
Dizziness
Fatigue

Insomnia
Palpitations
Poor digestion
Poor memory

Herbal prescription:

Ginseng *Ren Shen*	TQi	Angelica *Dang Gui*	TBl
Longan *Long Yan Rou*	TBl	Polygala *Yuan Zhi*	CS
Zizyphus *Suan Zao Ren*	CS	Saussurea *Mu Xiang*	RSQ
Poria *Fu Ling*	DD	Jujube *Da Zao*	TQi
Atractylodes *Bai Zhu*	TQi	Zingiberis *Sheng Jiang*	DWC
Astragalus *Huang Qi*	TQi	Glycerrhiza *Gan Cao*	TQi

Comments:

1. This formula is used for insomnia and palpitations due to deficiency of spleen *qi* and heart blood. Use **Ginseng & Zizyphus Formula** for insomnia due to deficiency of heart *yin* and blood.

Availability:

1. Zand Chinese Classics, McZand Herbal, Inc; herbal liquid extract.
2. As **Ginseng and Longan Combination**; extract granules.
3. As **Kwei Bi Wan**; Chinese patent medicine; pills.
4. As **Gather Vitality**; Jade Pharmacy, K'an Herb Company; herbal liquid extract or tablets.

28. GINSENG & TANG KUEI TEN FORMULA

Deficiency of qi and blood

Shi Quan Da Bu Tang
"Ten Inclusive Great Tonifying Decoction"

Energetic and functional presentation:

Deficiency of spleen *qi*
Deficiency of liver blood
Deficiency of spleen and kidney *yang*
Deficiency of *wei qi*
Deficiency of heart *qi* and *yang*

Tongue: Pale, swollen
Pulse: Weak, thin, soft

Symptoms and applications:

Amenorrhea	Palpitation
Anemia	Poor appetite
Cold limbs	Poor digestion
Dry skin	Post–partum
Fatigue	Post–surgery
Insomnia	Uterine bleeding
Irregular menstruation	Weak heart

Herbal prescription:

Angelica *Dang Gui*	TBI	Poria *Fu Ling*	DD
Rehmannia *Shu Di*	TBI	Glycerrhiza *Gan Cao*	TQi
Paeonia *Bai Shao*	TBI	Cinnamomum *Rou Gui*	WI
Ligusticum *Chuan Xiong*	IB	Astragalus *Huang Qi*	TQi
Codonopsis *Dang Shen*	TQi	Ginseng *Ren Shen*	TQi
Atractylodes *Bai Zhu*	TQi		

Availability:

1. Zand Chinese Classics, McZand Herbal, Inc; herbal liquid extract.
2. As **Ginseng and Tang–kuei Ten Combination**; extract granules.
3. As **Shi Chuan Da Bu Wan**; Chinese patent medicine; pills.

29. GINSENG & ZIZYPHUS FORMULA

Insomnia or palpitation due to deficiency of yin

Tian Wang Bu Xin Tang
"Heavenly Emperor Tonify Heart Decoction"

Energetic and functional presentation:

Deficiency of heart *yin*
Deficiency of heart blood
Deficiency of heart *qi*
Disturbed *shen*
Deficiency heat in the upper burner
Dysharmony of heart and kidney

Tongue: Red, dry
Pulse: Thin, rapid; may be irregular

Symptoms and applications:

Anxiety and nervousness
Hyperactive thyroid
Insomnia
Irregular pulse

Palpitation
Restlessness
Restless sleep

Herbal prescription:

Rehmannia *Sheng Di*	CBH	Ginseng *Ren Shen*	TQi
Scrophularia *Xuan Shen*	CBH	Biota *Bai Zi Ren*	CS
Schizandra *Wu Wei Zi*	AH	Polygala *Yuan Zhi*	CS
Asparagus *Tian Men Dong*	TYi	Poria *Fu Ling*	DD
Angelica *Dang Gui*	TBI	Salvia *Dan Shen*	IB
Ophiopogon *Mai Men Dong*	TYi	Platycodon *Jie Geng*	TPD
Zizyphus *Suan Zao Ren*	CS		

Comments:

1. This formula is preferred for insomnia due to deficiency of heart *yin*. For insomnia due to deficiency of heart blood, use **Ginseng & Longan Formula**.

Availability:

1. Zand Chinese Classics, McZand Herbal, Inc; herbal liquid extract.
2. As extract granules.
3. As **Emperor's Tea** or **Tien Wang Pu Hsin Wan**; Chinese patent medicine; pills.

30. GINSENG NUTRITIVE FORMULA

General tonic for the aged

Ren Shen Yang Rong Tang
"Ginseng Cultivate Luxurient Growth Decoction"

Energetic and functional presentation:

Deficiency spleen *qi*
Deficiency of heart *qi*
Deficiency of lung *qi*
Deficiency of heart *yang*
Deficiency of heart blood
Deficiency of liver blood
Disturbed *shen*
Dysharmony of heart and kidney

Tongue: Pale
Pulse: Weak, soft;
especially in spleen, heart or lung positions

Symptoms and applications:

Anxiety and nervousness
Chronic fatigue syndrome
Fatigue
General tonic for the aged
Insomnia
Irregular Pulse

Palpitation
Poor appetite
Postpartum fatigue
Post-surgery fatigue
Restless sleep

Herbal prescription:

Angelica *Dang Gui*	TBI	Citrus *Chen Pi*	RSQ
Rehmannia *Shu Di*	TBI	Schizandra *Wu Wei Zi*	AH
Paeonia *Bai Shao*	TBI	Polygala *Yuan Zhi*	CS
Atractylodes *Bai Zhu*	TQi	Glycerrhiza *Gan Cao*	TQi
Poria *Fu Ling*	DD	Zingiberis *Sheng Jiang*	DWC
Astragalus *Huang Qi*	TQi	Jujube *Da Zao*	TQi
Ginseng *Ren Shen*	TQi	Cinnamomum *Rou Gui*	WI

Comments:

1. A good general tonic for aging patients with concerns for a weak heart.

Availability:

1. Zand Chinese Classics, McZand Herbal, Inc; herbal liquid extract.
2. As **Ginseng Nutritive Combination**; extract granules.
3. As **Yang Rong Wan** (**Ginseng Tonic Pills**); Chinese patent medicine; pills.

31. GUAN JIE FORMULA
Rheumatoid arthritis
Guan Jie Yan Wan
"Close Down Joint Inflammation Pills"

Energetic and functional presentation:

Wind-damp-heat in the channels

Tongue: Occasionally red
Pulse: Weak, may be rapid; occasionally thin;
may be superficial

Symptoms and applications:

Hot, painful joints
Rheumatoid arthritis
Sciatic inflammation

Herbal prescription:

Erythrina *Hai Tong Pi*	DWD	Gentiana *Qin Jiao*	DWD
Phellodendron *Huang Bai*	CDH	Cinnamomum *Rou Gui*	WI
Atractylodes *Cang Zhu*	TSD	Zingiberis *Sheng Jiang*	DWC
Coix *Yi Yi Ren*	DD	Angelica *Du Huo*	DWD
Stephania *Hai Fang Ji*	DD	Ephedra *Ma Huang*	DWC
Achyranthes *Niu Xi*	TYi		

Comments:

1. Prohibited during pregnancy.
2. In heat conditions, it may be important to add boiling water to neutralize the heating effects of alcohol.

Availability:

1. Zand Chinese Classics, McZand Herbal, Inc; herbal liquid extract.
2. As **Guan Jie Yan Wan**; Chinese patent medicine; pills.

32. HOELEN FIVE FORMULA
Edema
Wu Ling San
"Five (Herb) Poria Powder"

Energetic and functional presentation:

Accumulation of damp
Deficiency of spleen *qi* with cold and damp
Wind-cold-damp accumulation

Tongue: Swollen, wet
Pulse: Wide, soft, slippery

Symptoms and applications:

Ascites
Diarrhea
Digestive disturbance due to
 cold and damp
Edema in limbs (mild)
Facial edema due to wind

Headache due to viral encephaly
Premenstrual bloating
Premenstrual water retention
Scrotal hydrocele
Urinary frequency
Urinary retention

Herbal prescription:

Alisma *Ze Xie*   DD   Atractylodes *Cang Zhu*   TQi
Poria *Fu Ling*   DD   Cinammomum *Gui Zhi*   DWC
Polyporous *Zhu Ling*   DD

Comments:

1. This formula acts as a mild diuretic, and can be valuable in a variety of situations.

Availability:

1. Zand Chinese Classics, McZand Herbal, Inc; herbal liquid extract.
2. As **Hoelen Five Herb Formula**; extract granules.

33. ISATIS FORMULA

Viral infections

Chuan Xin Lian Kang Yang Pian
"Andrographis Fight Heat Tablet"

Energetic and functional presentation:

Toxic heat in liver
Toxic heat in lung

Tongue: Red, or red in sides or upper third
Pulse: Excessive, rapid

Symptoms and applications:

Abscesses	Mumps
Chronic Fatigue Syndrome	Lymphatic congestion
Epstein–Barr Virus	Sore throat
Hepatitis	Strept throat
Herpes	Swollen liver
Influenza	Swollen lymph glands
Mastitis	Viral infections
Measles	Viral encephaly

Herbal prescription:

Isatis *Ban Lang Gen*	CTH	Arctium *Niu Bang Gen*	
Isatis *Da Qing Ye*	CTH	Viola *Zi Hua Di Ding*	CTH
Andrographis *Chuan Xin Lian*	CTH	Lithosperm *Zi Cao*	CBH
Taraxacum *Pu Gong Ying*	CTH	Prunella *Xia Ku Cao*	CIH
Arctium *Niu Bang Zi*	DWH		

Comments:

1. This product contains herbs with proven anti–viral effect. Can be used alone, or in conjunction with other formulas.
2. Excellent in infections producing sore throat and swollen lymph glands in the neck.
3. In heat conditions, it may be important to add boiling water to neutralize the heating effects of alcohol.

Availability:

1. Zand Chinese Classics, McZand Herbal, Inc; herbal liquid extract.

34. JADE SCREEN FORMULA
Tonify wei qi
Yu Ping Feng San
"Jade Screen Powder"

Energetic and functional presentation:

Deficiency of *wei qi*

Tongue: Normal
Pulse: Slightly weak in spleen or lung position

Symptoms and applications:

Desire to increase resistance to disease
Weak *wei qi* (defensive energy)

Herbal prescription:

Astragalus *Huang Qi*	TQi
Siler *Fang Feng*	DWC
Atractylodes *Bai Zhu*	TQi

Availability:

1. Zand Chinese Classics, McZand Herbal, Inc; herbal liquid extract.

35. JIN GU FORMULA

Traumatic injury

Jin Gu Die Shang Wan
"Muscles, Bone Traumatic Injury Pill"

Energetic and functional presentation:

Stagnation of *qi* and blood in channels

Tongue: May be purple or dark; or dark spots
Pulse: Choppy

Symptoms and applications:

Bone fractures	Post-surgical recovery
Bruises	Sprains with swelling
Dislocation of joints	Traumatic injury
Hemorrhoids	Wounds

Herbal prescription:

Pseudoginseng *Tian Qi*	SB		Dipsacus *Xu Duan*	TYa
Sanguis Draconis *Xue Jie*	IB		Drynaria *Gu Sui Bu*	TYa
Angelica *Dang Gui*	TBI		Curcuma *Yu Jin*	IB
Olibanum *Ru Xiang*	IB		Albizia *He Huan Pi*	IB
Myrrh *Mo Yao*	IB		Angelica *Bai Zhi*	DWC
Carthamus *Hong Hua*	IB		Amomum *Sha Ren*	TSD

Comments:

1. This formula offers excellent results for traumatic injury.
2. Prohibited during pregnancy.

Availability:

1. Zand Chinese Classics, McZand Herbal, Inc; herbal liquid extract.
2. As **Chin Koo Tieh Shang Wan**; Chinese patent medicine; pills.

36. LI DAN FORMULA
Gallstones or gallbladder inflammation
Li Dan Pian
"Benefit Gallbladder Tablets"

Energetic and functional presentation:

Gallbladder damp-heat
Stagnation of liver *qi* and blood
Toxic heat
Stagnation of stomach *qi* and damp

Tongue: May be swollen and/or pale;
Pulse: Weak, soft or slippery, especially in spleen position

Symptoms and applications:

Gallbladder inflammation
Gallstones
Hepatitis

Hepatomegaly
Roundworms in the biliary duct

Herbal prescription:

Lysimachia *Jin Qian Cao*	DD	Lonicera *Jin Yin Hua*	CTH
Scutellaria *Huang Qin*	CDH	Aurantium *Zhi Shi*	RSQ
Saussurea *Mu Xiang*	RSQ	Curcuma *Yu Jin*	IB
Artemesia *Yin Chen Hao*	DD	Magnolia *Hou Po*	TSD
Bupleurum *Chai Hu*	DWH	Areca *Da Fu Pi*	RSQ
Isatis *Da Qing Ye*	CTH	Rheum *Da Huang*	Pu

Comments:

1. This formula can dissolve gallstones, without a strong purgative effect. Caution should be made, however, for large stones, so as to avoid a surgical emergency. This is determined through ultrasound diagnosis.

Availability:

1. Zand Chinese Classics, McZand Herbal, Inc; herbal liquid extract.
2. Combines **Li Dan Tablets** and **Lidian Paishi Tablets**; Chinese patent medicine; pills.

37. LONGEVITY FORMULA
Deficiency of lung yin
Ba Xian Chang Shou Wan
"Eight Immortals Long Life Pill"

Energetic and functional presentation:

Deficiency of lung *yin*
Deficiency of kidney *yin*

Tongue: Dry coat; may be red, or red in tip
Pulse: Thin; weak in lung position

Symptoms and applications:

Afternoon low grade fever	Dry cough
	Dry mouth
Difficult breathing	Dry nose

Herbal prescription:

Rehmannia *Shu Di Huang*	TBI	Dioscorea *Shan Yao*		TQi
Ophiopogon *Mai Men Dong*	TYi	Poria *Fu Ling*		DD
Schizandra *Wu Wei Zi*	AH	Alisma *Ze Xie*		DD
Cornus *Shan Zhu Yu*	AH	Moutan *Mu Dan Pi*		CBH

Availability:

1. Zand Chinese Classics, McZand Herbal, Inc; herbal liquid extract.
2. As **Ba Xian Chang Shou Wan**; Chinese patent medicine; pills.

38. LYCIUM & REHMANNIA FORMULA

Deficiency of liver yin; Vision disorders

Qi Ju Di Huang Wan

"Lycium, Chrysanthemum, Rehmannia Pill"

Energetic and functional presentation:

Deficiency of liver *yin*
Deficiency of kidney *yin*

Tongue: Dry coat; may be red, or red on sides
Pulse: Thin, especially in liver position; may be rapid

Symptoms and applications:

Blurry vision	Glaucoma
Cataracts	Hypertension
Dizziness	Irregular menstruation
Dry eyes	Premenstrual syndrome

Herbal prescription:

Rehmannia *Shu Di Huang*	TBl	Alisma *Ze Xie*	DD
Cornus *Shan Zhu Yu*	AH	Moutan *Mu Dan Pi*	CBH
Dioscorea *Shan Yao*	TQi	Lycium *Gou Qi Zi*	TBl
Poria *Fu Ling*	DD	Chrysanthemum *Ju Hua*	DWH

Availability:

1. Zand Chinese Classics, McZand Herbal, Inc; herbal liquid extract.
2. As **Lycium, Chrysanthemum, and Rehmannia Formula**; extract granules.
3. As **Lycii and Chrysanthemum Tea**, and **Lycium–Rehmannia Pills**; Chinese patent medicine; pills.

39. MA HUANG & GINKGO PLUS FORMULA

Cough and asthma

Ding Chuan Tang
"Calm Asthma Decoction"

Energetic and functional presentation:

Wind–heat invasion to lung
Phlegm–heat in lung

Tongue: Red in upper third; thin or thick greasy yellow coat
Pulse: Wiry or tense in superficial level; may be slippery in deeper level; excessive in lung position

Symptoms and applications:

Asthma	Cough (rattling or wheezing)
Bronchitis	Difficulty breathing
Constriction of chest	Emphysema
Cough due to common cold	Yellow phlegm (sticky or copious)

Herbal prescription:

Ginkgo *Yin Guo*	AH	Gypsum *Shi Gao*	CIH
Ephedra *Ma Huang*	DWC	Tussilago *Kuan Dong Hua*	RCA
Perilla *Su Zi*	RCA	Pinellia *Ban Xia*	TPD
Armeniaca *Xing Ren*	RCA	Scutellaria *Huang Qin*	CDH
Morus *Sang Bai Pi*	RCA	Glycerrhiza *Gan Cao*	TQi

Comments:

1. Caution in products containing Ephedra; it may cause agitation in weaker patients, and insomnia in all patients.
2. Gypsum is added to enhance synergistic effect with Ephedra *Ma Huang*, allowing for relaxation of extrinsic and intrinsic muscles of the lung.

Availability:

1. Zand Chinese Classics, McZand Herbal, Inc; herbal liquid extract.
2. Without Gypsum, as **Ma–huang and Ginkgo Combination**; extract granules.

40. MINOR BLUE DRAGON FORMULA

Lung and watery nasal congestion

Xiao Qing Long Tang
"Minor Blue Dragon Decoction"

Energetic and functional presentation:

Wind–cold invasion into lungs
Accumulation of phlegm–damp in lung or nose
Deficiency of lung *qi*

Tongue: White, moist coat
Pulse: Weak–tense in the superficial level; or slippery

Symptoms and applications:

Asthma
Bronchitis
Common cold
Cough
Emphysema

Hayfever
Nasal congestion
Runny nose
Shortness of breath

Herbal prescription:

Pinellia *Ban Xia*	TPD	Zingiberis *Gan Jiang*	WI
Cinnamomum *Gui Zhi*	DWC	Ephedra *Ma Huang*	DWC
Paeonia *Bai Shao*	TBI	Asarum *Xi Xin*	DWC
Schizandra *Wu Wei Zi*	AH	Glycerrhiza *Gan Cao*	TQi

Comments:

1. Caution in products containing Ephedra; it may cause agitation in weaker patients, and insomnia in all patients.
2. This formula is preferred for copious watery phlegm, in lung or nose.

Availability:

1. Zand Chinese Classics, McZand Herbal, Inc; herbal liquid extract.
2. As **Minor Blue Dragon Combination**; extract granules.
3. As **Minor Blue Dragon**; Health Concerns; tablets.

41. MINOR BUPLEURUM FORMULA

Chronic disorders

Xiao Chai Hu Tang
"Minor Bupleurum Decoction"

Energetic and functional presentation:

Dysharmony of liver and spleen
Liver *qi* stagnation
Dysharmony of interior and exterior
Stagnation of *qi* in the GB channel
Accumulation of phlegm in stomach
Deficiency of spleen *qi*
Liver heat

Tongue: Red on sides; yellow coat
Pulse: Wiry in gallbladder, liver and stomach positions;
weak in spleen position

Symptoms and applications:

Alternating chills and fevers	Muscular tension in neck and shoulders
Anxiety	Poor appetite
Chronic hepatitis	Poor sleep
Epigastric distension	Prolonged cold or flu
Headache	Restlessness
Hypoglycemia	Smoking and drug withdrawal

Herbal prescription:

Bupleurum *Chai Hu*	DWH	Codonopsis *Dang Shen*	TQi
Pinellia *Ban Xia*	TPD	Jujube *Da Zao*	TQi
Zingiberis *Sheng Jiang*	DWC	Glycerrhiza *Gan Cao*	TQi
Scutellaria *Huang Qin*	CDH		

Comments:

1. Bupleurum formulas may open and invigorate the liver too quickly, causing side effects of symptom aggravation, digestive problems, or irritability. If this is the case, reduce dosage.

Availability:

1. Zand Chinese Classics, McZand Herbal, Inc; herbal liquid extract.
2. As **Minor Bupleurum Combination**; extract granules.

42. OPHIOPOGON & ASARUM FORMULA

Headache

Qing Shang Juan Tong Tang
"Clear Upper, Remove Pain Decoction"

Energetic and functional presentation:

Stagnation of wind–cold–damp in the channels
Stagnation of *qi* and blood in the channels
Liver and gallbladder heat

Tongue: Red on sides; possibly swollen
Pulse: Tense, wiry or choppy in superficial level;
wiry in liver and gallbladder positions

Symptoms and applications:

Headache
Headache due to common
   cold
Migraine
Neck and shoulder tension

Sinus congestion
Sinus headache
Temporal–mandibular joint
   pain (TMJ)
Trigeminal neuralgia

Herbal prescription:

Scutellaria *Huang Qin*	CDH	Atractylodes *Bai Zhu*	TQi
Siler *Fang Feng*	DWC	Chrysanthemum *Ju Hua*	DWH
Ophiopogon *Mai Men Dong*	TYi	Vitex *Man Jing Zi*	DWH
Angelica *Du Huo*	DWD	Zingiberis *Sheng Jiang*	DWC
Angelica *Dang Gui*	TBI	Glycerrhiza *Gan Cao*	TQi
Ligusticum *Chuan Xiong*	IB	Asarum *Xi Xin*	DWC
Notopterygium *Qiang Huo*	DWC		

Availability:

1. Zand Chinese Classics, McZand Herbal, Inc; herbal liquid extract.
2. As **Ophiopogon and Asarum Combination**; extract granules.

43. OPHIOPOGON PLUS FORMULA

Deficient yin in lungs and stomach; Dry cough

Sha Shen Mai Men Dong Tang
"Glehnia, Ophiopogon Decoction

Energetic and functional presentation:

Deficiency of lung *yin* with heat
Deficiency of stomach *yin*

Tongue: Whole tongue glossy red, or red in upper third (tip);
red along midline; dry coat
Pulse: Thin, weak, slightly rapid

Symptoms and applications:

Cough following flu or cold	Fatigue
Dry cough	Sticky, hard to expectorate
Dry lips, mouth, nose	phlegm
Dry stools or constipation	Thirst
Dry throat	

Herbal prescription:

Ophiopogon *Mai Men Dong*	TYi	Pinellia *Ban Xia*	TPD
Codonopsis *Dang Shen*	TQi	Quinquefolium *Xi Yang Shen*	TYi
Glehnia *Bei Sha Shen*	TYi	Armeniaca *Xing Ren*	RCA
Polygonatum *Yu Zhu*	TYi	Morus *Sang Ye*	DWH
Asparagus *Tian Men Dong*	TYi	Morus *Sang Bai Pi*	RCA
Dendrobrium *Shi Hu*	TYi	Jujube *Da Zao*	TQi
Trichosanthes *Tian Hua Fen*	TPH	Glycerrhiza *Gan Cao*	TQi
Platycodon *Jie Geng*	TPD		

Availability:

1. Zand Chinese Classics, McZand Herbal, Inc; herbal liquid extract.
2. As the combination of **Ophiopogon Combination** and **Adenophora and Ophiopogon Combination**; extract granules.

44. PASSWAN FORMULA
Kidney stones
Te Xiao Pai Shi Wan
"Specially Effective Discharge Stone Pill"

Energetic and functional presentation:

Kidney damp-heat
Urinary bladder damp-heat

Tongue: Raised red thorns in back;
thin yellow greasy coat in back
Pulse: Occasionally excessive in kidney positions (proximal third)

Symptoms and applications:

Hematuria	Kidney stone
Kidney infection	Urinary bladder stone
Kidney inflammation	

Herbal prescription:

Lysimachia *Jin Qian Cao*	DD	Coptis *Huang Lian*	CDH
Lygodium *Hai Jin Sha*	CTH	Milettia *Ji Xue Teng*	IB
Angelica *Bai Zhi*	DWC	Rheum *Da Huang*	Pu
Andrographis *Chuan Xin Lian*	CTH	Pseudoginseng *Tian Qi*	SB
Cyathula *Chuan Niu Xi*	IB	Succinum *Hu Po*	CS

Comments:

1. This formula will work to dissolve kidney stones. Not effective for acute attack, it is best used in chronic conditions, or people susceptible to repeat attacks. Use for one to two months.
2. Acute obstruction requires use of other modalities, such as hot compresses, electro-acupuncture, or surgery.

Availability:

1. Zand Chinese Classics, McZand Herbal, Inc; herbal liquid extract.
2. As **Specific Drug Passwan**; Chinese patent medicine; pills.

45. PINELLIA & MAGNOLIA FORMULA

Nausea; Chronic phlegm

Ban Xia Hou Po Tang

"Pinellia, Magnolia Decoction"

Energetic and functional presentation:

Accumulation of damp and phlegm in the stomach
Stagnation of stomach qi

Tongue: Swollen, wet; greasy white or yellow coating
Pulse: Soft or slippery; occasionally wiry; weak in spleen position

Symptoms and applications:

Cough due to lung phlegm
Epigastric distension
Food poisoning
Food stagnation
Globus hystericus

Morning sickness
Nausea
Plum–pit in throat
Poor appetitie
Vomiting

Herbal prescription:

Pinellia *Ban Xia*	TPD	Zingiberis *Sheng Jiang*	DWC
Poria *Fu Ling*	DD	Perilla *Zi Su Ye*	DWC
Magnolia *Hou Po*	TSD		

Availability:

1. Zand Chinese Classics, McZand Herbal, Inc; herbal liquid extract.
2. As **Pinellia and Magnolia Combination**; extract granules.

46. PINELLIA "X" FORMULA

Lung phlegm–damp

Qing Qi Hua Tan Wan
"Clear Qi, Expel Phlegm Pill"

Energetic and functional presentation:

Lung phlegm–damp
Lung phlegm-heat

Tongue: Wet, white to grey coat
Pulse: Slippery; excess in lung position

Symptoms and applications:

Asthma, chronic
Cough with white or clear
  phlegm
Emphysema

Oppression in the chest
Pneumonia, chronic
Sinus phlegm

Herbal prescription:

Pinellia *Ban Xia Tian*	TPD	Poria *Fu Ling*	DD
Arisaema *Nan Xing*	TPD	Trichosanthes *Gua Lou Ren*	TPH
Citrus *Chen Pi*	RSQ	Scutellaria*Huang Qin*	CDH
Armeniaca *Xing Ren*	RCA	Aurantium *Zhi Shi*	RSQ

Availability:

1. Zand Chinese Classics, McZand Herbal, Inc; herbal liquid extract.
2. As **Pinellia Expectorant Pills** or **Clean Air Tea**; Chinese patent medicine; pills.

47. PLATYCODON & FRITILLARIA FORMULA

Cough with sticky phlegm-heat

Qing Fei Tang
"Clear Lung Decoction"

Energetic and functional presentation:

Deficiency of lung *yin* with heat
Accumulation of lung phlegm-heat
Deficiency of lung *qi*

Tongue: Red, or red upper third; thin dry yellow coat
Pulse: Thin, slightly rapid;
excessive in lung position

Symptoms and applications:

Bronchitis
Dry cough with small,
scanty yellow phlegm

Emphysema
Smoker's cough

Herbal prescription:

Platycodon *Jie Geng*	TPD	Bambusa *Zhu Ru*	TPH
Fritillaria *Chuan Bei Mu*	TPH	Gardenia *Zhi Zi*	CIH
Ophiopogon *Mai Men Dong*	TYi	Citrus *Chen Pi*	RSQ
Poria *Fu Ling*	DD	Schizandra *Wu Wei Zi*	AH
Jujube *Da Zao*	TQi	Morus *Sang Bai Pi*	RCA
Angelica *Dang Gui*	TBI	Asparagus *Tian Men Dong*	TYi
Scutellaria *Huang Qin*	CDH	Zingiberis *Sheng Jiang*	DWC
Armeniaca *Xing Ren*	RCA	Glycerrhiza *Gan Cao*	TQi

Availability:

1. Zand Chinese Classics, McZand Herbal, Inc; herbal liquid extract.
2. As **Platycodon and Fritillaria Combination**; extract granules.

48. PUERARIA FORMULA
Common cold
Ge Gen Tang
"Pueraria Decoction"

Energetic and functional presentation:

Wind–cold invasion
Constriction of gallbladder channel

Tongue: Normal
Pulse: Tense and forceful in superficial position;
may be excess in gallbladder position

Symptoms and applications:

Asthma, chronic
Common cold
Difficult breathing

Headache due to wind
invasion
Stiff neck and shoulders

Herbal prescription:

Pueraria *Ge Gen*	DWH	Jujube *Da Zao*	TQi
Ephedra *Ma Huang*	DWC	Glycerrhiza *Gan Cao*	TQi
Cinnamomum *Gui Zhi*	DWC	Zingiberis *Sheng Jiang*	DWC
Paeonia *Bai Shao*	TBI		

Comments:

1. This formula can act as an herbal vasodilator in asthmatic constriction of the lungs.

Availability:

1. Zand Chinese Classics, McZand Herbal, Inc; herbal liquid extract.
2. As **Pueraria Combination**; extract granules.

49. PUERARIA "N" FORMULA
Nasal and sinus congestion
Qing Bi Tang
"Clear Nose Decoction"

Energetic and functional presentation:

Wind–cold invasion to lung
Lung phlegm–heat
Heat in the lung, large intestine and stomach channels
Lung phlegm–damp

Tongue: Red in upper third and along midline; yellow coating
Pulse: Superficial, occasionally slippery; may be rapid;
excessive in distal third (upper burner)

Symptoms and applications:

Earaches	Sinus headache
Rhinitis	Snoring
Sinus congestion	Thick nasal discharge

Herbal prescription:

Pueraria *Ge Gen*	DWH	Gypsum *Shi Gao*	CIH
Magnolia *Xin Yi Hua*	DWC	Jujube *Da Zao*	TQi
Coix *Yi Yi Ren*	DD	Zingiberis *Sheng Jiang*	DWC
Platycodon *Jie Geng*	TPD	Rheum *Da Huang*	Pu
Paeonia *Bai Shao*	TBI	Ligusticum *Chuan Xiong*	IB
Ephedra *Ma Huang*	DWC	Glycerrhiza *Gan Cao*	TQi
Cinnamomum *Gui Zhi*	DWC		

Comments:

1. In chronic sinus congestion or hayfever, evaluate liver, gallbladder, and stomach/spleen functions.

Availability:

1. Zand Chinese Classics, McZand Herbal, Inc; herbal liquid extract.
2. As **Pueraria Nasal Combination**; extract granules.
3. As **Nasal Combination**; Health Concerns; tablets.

50. REHMANNIA EIGHT PLUS FORMULA

Deficiency of kidney yang

Jin Kui Shen Qi Jia Wan
"Golden Deficient Kidney *Qi* (Plus) Pills"

Energetic and functional presentation:

Deficiency of kidney *yang*

Tongue: Pale, or normal
Pulse: Weak in kidney positions (proximal third)

Symptoms and applications:

Chronic lower back problems	Loose stools
Cold limbs	Weak or cold knees
Cold torso	Weak or cold lower back
Diabetes	

Herbal prescription:

Eucommia *Du Zhong*	TYa	Cinnamomum *Rou Gui*	WI
Rehmannia *Shu Di Huang*	TBl	Morinda *Ba Ji Tian*	TYa
Cornus *Shan Zhu Yu*	AH	Cistanche *Rou Cong Rong*	TYa
Dioscorea *Shan Yao*	TQi	Cynomorium *Suo Yang*	TYa
Poria *Fu Ling*	DD	Psoralea *Bu Gu Zhi*	TYa
Alisma *Ze Xie*	DD	Cuscuta *Tu Si Zi*	TYa
Moutan *Mu Dan Pi*	CBH	Lycium *Gou Qi Zi*	TBl

Availability:

1. Zand Chinese Classics, McZand Herbal, Inc; herbal liquid extract.

51. REHMANNIA SIX FORMULA

Deficiency of kidney yin

Liu Wei Di Huang Wan
"Six Flavor Rehmannia Pill"

Energetic and functional presentation:

Deficiency of kidney *yin*
Deficiency of liver *yin*
Deficiency of stomach *yin*

Tongue: Thin body; dry coat
Pulse: Thin; occasionally slightly rapid

Symptoms and applications:

Dry eyes	Fatigue
Dry mouth	Thirst
Dry stools or constipation	Weak lower back

Herbal prescription:

Rehmannia *Shu Di Huang*	TBI	Poria *Fu Ling*	DD
Cornus *Shan Zhu Yu*	AH	Alisma *Ze Xie*	DD
Dioscorea *Shan Yao*	TQi	Moutan *Mu Dan Pi*	CBH

Availability:

1. Zand Chinese Classics, McZand Herbal, Inc; herbal liquid extract.
2. As extract granules.
3. As **Six Flavor Tea** or **Liu Wei Di Huang Wan**; Chinese patent medicine; pills.

52. SALVIA PLUS FORMULA
Heart blood stagnation; Elevated cholesterol
Dan Shen Yin
"Salvia Cool Decoction"

Energetic and functional presentation:

Blood stagnation in the heart and channels
Stagnation of liver blood

Tongue: May be dark or purple, or purple spots
Pulse: Choppy; excess in heart position

Symptoms and applications:

Angina	Elevated blood cholesterol and lipids
Chest pain	Heart attack
Chronic hepatitis	High blood pressure
Difficulty breathing	Stroke

Herbal prescription:

Salvia *Dan Shen*	IB	Angelica *Dang Gui*	TBI
Polygonum *He Shou Wu*	TBI	Schizandra *Wu Wei Zi*	AH
Morus *Sang Shen*	TBI	Paeonia *Chi Shao*	IB
Crataegus *Shan Zha*	RFS	Scutellaria *Huang Qin*	CDH
Cassia *Jue Ming Zi*	CIH	Santalum *Tan Xiang*	RSQ
Alisma *Ze Xie*	DD	Amomum *Sha Ren*	TSD
Eucommia *Du Zhong*	TYa	Saussurea *Mu Xiang*	RSQ

Comments:

1. This formula includes many of the proven anti–blood lipid herbs in the Chinese materia medica. It also contains a number of herbs known to lower high blood pressure. It is a good preventative against heart attack and stroke.

Availability:

1. Zand Chinese Classics, McZand Herbal, Inc; herbal liquid extract.

53. SAUSSUREA & CARDAMON FORMULA

Digestive disorders due to spleen qi deficiency

Xiang Sha Liu Jun Zi Tang
"Saussurea, Amomum, Six Gentlemen Decoction"

Energetic and functional presentation:

Deficiency of spleen *qi*
Accumulation of stomach phlegm-damp
Stagnation of stomach *qi*

Tongue: May be swollen and/or pale;
thin white greasy coat
Pulse: Weak, soft or slippery, especially in spleen position

Symptoms and applications:

Abdominal distension	Loose stools
Fatigue	Morning sickness
Gas or flatulence	Nausea
Food stagnation	Poor appetite
Indigestion	

Herbal prescription:

Atractylodes *Bai Zhu*	TQi	Saussurea *Mu Xiang*	RSQ
Poria *Fu Ling*	DD	Amomum *Sha Ren*	TSD
Pinellia *Ban Xia*	TPD	Glycerrhiza *Zhi Gan Cao*	TQi
Codonopsis *Dang Shen*	TQi	Ginseng *Ren Shen*	TQi
Citrus *Chen Pi*	RSQ	Zingiberis *Sheng Jiang*	DWC

Comments:

1. This is one of the best tonics for spleen *qi* deficiency.
2. Excellent for morning sickness due to spleen *qi* deficiency.
3. The herb "Cardamon" is listed as Amomum *Sha Ren*.

Availability:

1. Zand Chinese Classics, McZand Herbal, Inc; herbal liquid extract.
2. As **Saussurea and Cardamon Combination**; extract granules.
3. As **Aplotaxis-Amomum Pills**; **Hsiang Sha Liu Jun Zi Wan**; or **Six Gentlemen Tea Pill**; Chinese patent medicine; pills.

54. SHOU WU FORMULA
Blood & jing deficiency
Shou Wu Zhi
"Polygonum He Shou Wu Juice"

Energetic and functional presentation:

Deficiency of liver blood
Deficiency of *jing*
Deficiency of liver *yin*
Stagnation of blood

Tongue: Pale
Pulse: Weak or thin

Symptoms and applications:

Amenorrhea
Blurry vision
Dizziness
Dry or brittle hair
Dry skin
Dry throat or lungs
Elevated blood cholesterol
   and fats

Fatigue
Insomnia
Late or scanty periods
Post-fever fatigue or dryness
Post-partum fatigue
Post-surgical fatigue
Sexual exhaustion in men
Spots in vision

Herbal prescription:

Polygonum *He Shou Wu*	TBI	Ligusticum *Chuan Xiong*	IB
Angelica *Dang Gui*	TBI	Angelica *Bai Zhi*	DWC
Polygonatum *Huang Jing*	TQi	Amomum *Sha Ren*	TSD
Rehmannia *Shu Di Huang*	TBI	Caryophyllum *Ding Xiang*	WI
Paeonia *Bai Shao*	TBI	Citrus *Chen Pi*	RSQ

Availability:

1. Zand Chinese Classics, McZand Herbal, Inc; herbal liquid extract.
2. As **Shou Wu Chih**; Chinese patent medicine; liquid extract.

55. SHU KAN FORMULA

Liver–stomach imbalance

Shu Gan Wan
"Comfort Liver Pills"

Energetic and functional presentation:

Stagnation of liver *qi*
Stagnation of stomach *qi*

Tongue: Normal, or thin greasy coat
Pulse: Excess or wiry in liver and stomach positions

Symptoms and applications:

Belching
Costal distension of pain
Epigastric distension
Epigastric pain
Flatulence

Hiccup
Hypoglycemia
Poor appetite
Poor digestion

Herbal prescription:

Cyperus *Xiang Fu*	RSQ	Inula *Xuan Fu Hua*	TPD
Paeonia *Bai Shao*	TBI	Glycerrhiza *Gan Cao*	TQi
Citrus *Chen Pi*	RSQ	Curcuma *Yu Jin*	IB
Citrus *Qing Pi*	RSQ	Amomum *Bai Dou Kou*	TSD
Corydalis *Yan Hu Suo*	IB	Aquilaria *Chen Xiang*	RSQ
Bupleurum *Chai Hu*	DWH	Magnolia *Hou Po*	TSD
Aurantium *Zhi Ke*	RSQ	Saussurea *Mu Xiang*	RSQ
Amomum *Sha Ren*	TSD	Santalum *Tan Xiang*	RSQ
Moutan *Mu Dan Pi*	CBH		

Availability:

1. Zand Chinese Classics, McZand Herbal, Inc; herbal liquid extract.
2. As **Shu Kan Wan**; Chinese patent medicine; pills.

56. SILER & PLATYCODON FORMULA

Fever with constipation during common cold or flu

Fang Feng Tong Sheng Tang
"Siler Opened (by the) Sage Decoction"

Energetic and functional presentation:

Heat in the *yangming* (stomach and intestines)
Invasion of wind
Toxic heat
Heat in the liver

Tongue: Red; dry or yellow coating
Pulse: Superficial and deep, forceful, rapid

Symptoms and applications:

Aching limbs	Flu
Acute constipation	High fever in common cold

Herbal prescription:

Talcum *Hua Shi*	DD	Mirabilite *Mang Xiao*	Pu
Gypsum *Shi Gao*	CIH	Angelica *Dang Gui*	TBI
Platycodon *Jie Geng*	TPH	Ligusticum *Chuan Xiong*	IB
Atractylodes *Bai Zhu*	TQi	Rheum *Da Huang*	Pu
Paeonia *Bai Shao*	TBI	Ephedra *Ma Huang*	DWC
Siler *Fang Feng*	DWC	Gardenia *Zhi Zi*	CIH
Scutellaria *Huang Qin*	CDH	Zingiberis *Sheng Jiang*	DWC
Forsythia *Lian Qiao*	CTH	Mentha *Bo He*	DWH
Schizonepeta *Jing Jie*	DWC	Glycerrhiza *Gan Cao*	TQi

Comments:

1. Do not use if there are loose stools. Discontinue or reduce dosage if diarrhea develops.
2. This formula has been used for obesity in cases characterized by stagnation-heat, with constipation.

Availability:

1. Zand Chinese Classics, McZand Herbal, Inc; herbal liquid extract.
2. As **Siler and Platycodon Combination**; extract granules.

57. TANG KUEI & ARCTIUM FORMULA

Skin disorders

Xiao Feng San
"Dispel Wind Powder"

Energetic and functional presentation:

Wind-blood-heat on the surface

Tongue: Red, or red on sides and upper third
Pulse: Superficial, slightly rapid

Symptoms and applications:

Acne	Itching
Dermatitis	Prickly heat
Eczema	Pruritis
Hives	Rash

Herbal prescription:

Angelica *Dang Gui*	TBl	Sesame *He Zhi Ma*	TYi
Rehmannia *Sheng Di Huang*	CBH	Anemarrhena *Zhi Mu*	CIH
Gypsum *Shi Gao*	CIH	Schizonepeta *Jing Jie*	DWC
Arctium *Niu Bang Zi*	DWH	Sophora *Ku Shen*	CDH
Akebia *Mu Tong*	DD	Cicada *Chan Tui*	DWH
Atractylodes *Cang Zhu*	TQi	Glycerrhiza *Gan Cao*	TQi
Siler *Fang Feng*	DWC		

Comments:

1. Use for skin conditions characterized by redness, rash, or itching.
2. In heat conditions, it may be important to add boiling water to neutralize the heating effects of alcohol.

Availability:

1. Zand Chinese Classics, McZand Herbal, Inc; herbal liquid extract.
2. As extract granules.

58. TANG KUEI & GINSENG EIGHT FORMULA

Deficiency of qi and blood

Ba Zhen Tang
"Eight Treasure Decoction"

Energetic and functional presentation:

Deficiency of spleen *qi*
Deficiency of liver blood

Tongue: Pale; may be swollen
Pulse: Thin, weak

Symptoms and applications:

Amenorrhea
Anemia
Delayed menses
Dizziness
Dry or brittle hair
Dry skin
Fatigue

Fatigue following prolonged illness
Irregular menses
Loose stools
Poor digestion
Post-menstrual fatigue
Post-partum fatigue
Spots in vision

Herbal prescription:

Angelica *Dang Gui*	TBl	Poria *Fu Ling*	DD
Rehmannia *Shu Di Huang*	TBl	Ligusticum *Chuan Xiong*	IB
Paeonia *Bai Shao*	TBl	Glycerrhiza *Gan Cao*	TQi
Codonopsis *Dang Shen*	TQi	Ginseng *Ren Shen*	TQi
Atractylodes *Bai Zhu*	TQi		

Availability:

1. Zand Chinese Classics, McZand Herbal, Inc; herbal liquid extract.
2. As **Tang-kuei and Ginseng Eight Combination**; extract granules.
3. As **Eight Treasure Tea** or **Women's Precious Pills**; Chinese patent medicine; pills.

59. TANG KUEI & PEONY FORMULA

Premenstrual water retention; Abdominal pain during pregnancy

Dang Gui Shao Yao Tang
"Angelica *Dang Gui*, Paeonia *Bai Shao* Decoction"

Energetic and functional presentation:

Water retention in the lower burner
Deficiency of blood
Deficiency of kidney *qi*

Tongue: Pale or normal
Pulse: Slightly slippery; may also be wiry

Symptoms and applications:

Abdominal pain during
   pregnancy
Habitual miscarriage
Infertility

Lower back pain
Post-partum fatigue
Premenstrual water retention

Herbal prescription:

Paeonia *Bai Shao*	TBI	Alisma *Ze Xie*	DD
Poria *Fu Ling*	DD	Angelica *Dang Gui*	TBI
Atractylodes *Bai Zhu*	TQi	Ligusticum *Chuan Xiong*	IB

Comments:

1. Chinese herbal medicine should be given during pregnancy only by experienced and well trained practitioners. Numerous sources cite Ligusticum *Chuan Xiong* as contraindicated during pregnancy.

Availability:

1. Zand Chinese Classics, McZand Herbal, Inc; herbal liquid extract.
2. As extract granules.

60. TANG KUEI FOUR FORMULA
Blood deficiency
Si Wu Tang
"Four Substance Decoction"

Energetic and functional presentation:
Deficiency of blood

Tongue: Pale
Pulse: Thin and weak

Symptoms and applications:

Amenorrhea	Fatigue
Anemia	Irregular menses
Constipation	Poor nails
Delayed menses	Post-menstrual fatigue
Dry or brittle hair	Spots in vision
Dry skin	

Herbal prescription:

Angelica *Dang Gui*	TBI	Paeonia *Bai Shao*	TBI
Rehmannia *Shu Di Huang*	TBI	Ligusticum *Chuan Xiong*	IB

Comments:
1. For best results, combine with a *qi* tonic, such as **Four Gentlemen Formula**.

Availability:
1. Zand Chinese Classics, McZand Herbal, Inc; herbal liquid extract.
2. As **Tang–kuei Four Combination**; extract granules.

61. TO JING FORMULA

Menstrual cramping

Tong Jing Wan
"Regulate Menses Pill"

Energetic and functional presentation:

Stagnation of blood in uterus
Stagnation of liver blood

Tongue: Dark or purple; or purple spots
Pulse: Choppy

Symptoms and applications:

Ovarian cyst   Menstrual pain
Menstrual clots   Uterine fibroids
Menstrual cramps

Herbal prescription:

Curcuma *Yu Jin*	IB	Ligusticum *Chuan Xiong*	IB
Sparganium *San Leng*	IB	Angelica *Dang Gui*	TBI
Paeonia *Chi Shao*	IB	Salvia *Dan Shen*	IB
Carthamus *Hong Hua*	IB		

Comments:

1. This formula can be taken 2–3 days prior to the period, or throughout the month.
2. Increase formula during days of heavy cramping.

Availability:

1. Zand Chinese Classics, McZand Herbal, Inc; herbal liquid extract.
2. As **To Jing Wan**; Chinese patent medicine; pills.

62. YIN QIAO FORMULA
Wind–heat invasion (common cold)
Yin Qiao San
"Lonicera, Forsythia Powder"

Energetic and functional presentation:
Invasion of toxic wind-heat

Tongue: Normal; may be red in the upper third
Pulse: Forceful, superficial, rapid

Symptoms and applications:

Aching shoulders and neck
Common cold
Flu
Measles
Restless sleep

Sinus congestion
Slight fever
Sore throat
Swollen lymph glands
Tonsillitis

Herbal prescription:

Lonicera *Jin Yin Hua*	CTH	Phragmites *Lu Gen*	CIH
Forsythia *Lian Qiao*	CTH	Bambusa *Zhu Ye*	TPH
Soja *Dan Dou Shi*	DWH	Schizonepeta *Jing Jie*	DWC
Platycodon *Jie Geng*	TPD	Mentha *Bo He*	DWH
Arctium *Niu Bang Zi*	DWH	Glycerrhiza *Gan Cao*	TQi

Comments:
1. This formula is most effective when taken during the first 24 hours of the invasion. It is appropriate when sore throat is the main symptom.
2. Lonicera and Forsythia have strong effect against respiratory viruses.
3. It is advisable to increase dosage to 3-5 droppers every 2 hours.
4. Certain clinicians feel that this formula is effective in wind-cold invasions as well.

Availability:
1. Zand Chinese Classics, McZand Herbal, Inc; herbal liquid extract.
2. As **Lonicera and Forsythia Formula**; extract granules.
3. Similar to **Yinchiao Chieh Tu Pien**; Chinese patent medicine; pills.

63. ZHONG GAN LING FORMULA

Strong flu with fever

Zhong Gan Ling
"Valuable Cold Efficacious-Remedy"

Energetic and functional presentation:

Invasion of toxic wind-heat
Internal heat

Tongue: Red in upper third, or whole tongue red
Pulse: Superficial and excessive

Symptoms and applications:

Aching neck and shoulders
Common cold
Cough
Fever
Flu

Headache due to cold or flu
Sore throat
Strept throat
Swollen glands

Herbal prescription:

Ilex *Mao Dong Qing*	CTH	Artemesia *Qing Hao*	CSH
Pueraria *Ge Gen*	DWH	Gypsum *Shi Gao*	CIH
Verbena *Ma Bian Cao*	CTH	Notopterygium *Qiang Huo*	DWC
Isatis *Ban Lang Gen*	CTH		

Comments:

1. Use for strong flu with fever and aching neck and shoulders.
2. It is advisable to increase dosage to 3-5 droppers every 2 hours.
3. Effective in bacterial strept throat or bronchitis.
4. Verbena *Ma Bian Cao* is contraindicated during pregnancy.
5. In heat conditions, it may be important to add boiling water to neutralize the heating effects of alcohol.

Availability:

1. Zand Chinese Classics, McZand Herbal, Inc; herbal liquid extract.
2. As **Zhong Gan Ling**; Chinese patent medicine; pills.

64. ZIZYPHUS FORMULA
Insomnia due to deficiency heat
Suan Zao Ren Tang
"Zizyphus Decoction"

Energetic and functional presentation:

Deficiency of heart blood
Deficiency of heart yin with heat
Deficiency of liver blood
Stagnation of heart blood

Tongue: Pale; red in upper third; dry coating
Pulse: Thin, slightly rapid; may be choppy
slight excess in heart position

Symptoms and applications:

Dizziness
Insomnia
Night sweat (mild)

Palpitation
Restless sleep
Tachycardia

Herbal prescription:

Zizyphus *Suan Zao Ren* CS
Poria *Fu Shen* DD
Ligusticum *Chuan Xiong* IB

Anemarrhena *Zhi Mu* CIH
Glycerrhiza *Gan Cao* TQi

Availability:

1. Zand Chinese Classics, McZand Herbal, Inc; herbal liquid extract.
2. As **Zizyphus Combination**; extract granules.

GLOSSARY OF
TRADITIONAL CHINESE MEDICAL TERMS

BLOOD HEAT...A pathology where the blood heats up due to liver or heart fire, or systemic fever. The main symptom is non-traumatic bleeding, including nosebleed, uterine bleeding, and internal hemorrhaging, including rashes.

BLOOD STAGNATION...A condition where the blood congeals, moves slowly, or forms clots. Due to cold, heat, deficiency or trauma.

BURNERS...The upper burner is the area above the diaphragm and includes the lungs, heart and head; the middle burner is the area between the diaphragm and the naval, and includes the organs stomach, spleen, liver and gallbladder. It often relates to digestion in general. The lower burner is below the naval, and includes the kidneys, bladder, small and large intestines, uterus and genital organs. It also includes the liver and gallbladder channels.

CENTER...can refer to either the middle burner in general, or the stomach and spleen specifically.

DAMP...refers to exogenous invasion affecting the musculo-skeletal system (wind-damp), or endogenous weakness of the spleen leading to watery accumulations in organs or cavities.

DAMP-HEAT ...A pathological condition combining both excess damp and excess heat. It can affect the liver, gallbladder, intestines or uterus.

DEFICIENCY-HEAT...Excess heat which has its basis in deficiency of *yin*. It can affect the body systemically or appear isolated in the lungs, heart, stomach-spleen, liver, or kidneys.

EXOGENOUS INVASION...Any sickness whose origin is outside the body; includes wind invasions (colds), and toxic invasions (bacterial and viral) including measles, flu, encephalitis, meningitis, etc.

JING...Condensed essence of prenatal *qi* which is stored in the kidneys and circulates in the Eight Extra Channels. Related to sperm and ova production, as well as nurturing the fetus. Provides the basis for strong or weak constitutions.

LIVER FIRE...Pathological fever in the liver, with symptoms rising upwards to include headache, eye burning, ear-ringing, and insomnia.

PHLEGM...Congealed mucus formed by excesses of damp and heat. Often originates in the spleen and stomach due to heat in the gallbladder or liver, and accumulates in the lungs, sinuses, intestines, uterus, or the acupuncture channels. Includes fatty deposits in the heart and blood vessels.

PHLEGM-DAMP...Chronic phlegm which is clear or white, and affects primarily the lungs, heart, breast, uterus or digestive tract. Distinguished from phlegm-heat.

PHLEGM-HEAT...Acute phlegm, yellow and odorous, found primarily in the lungs, sinuses, stomach or uterus.

PULSES...ABNORMAL:
Choppy - width and height vary in volume (between thin and wide, excess and weak), although the rate is constant. Indicates blood stagnation.
Excess (forceful) - height of pulse is strong, forceful and hard. Indicates excess or stagnation of *qi*.
Irregular - rate is not constant. Includes speeding and slowing, regular missed beat, or irregular missed beat. Indicates congenital or acquired pathology of the heart, including stagnation of blood or phlegm, or deficiency of heart *qi*, *yang*, *yin*, or blood.
Rapid - the rate is greater than seventy-five beats per minute. Indicates heat, either deficiency or excess.
Slippery - a wide pulse, feeling full of oil or water. Indicates accumulation of damp or phlegm. Commonly seen in obese people, and pregnancy during the last trimester.
Soft - a weak pulse, which may be thin or wide. Indicates deficiency of *qi*, or *qi* and blood.
Superficial - of the three depths of the pulse, indicates a problem on the surface, such as wind invasion or skin problem, or a problem in the channels of the extremities.
Tense - refers to **wiry** or **tight** pulses.
Thin - refers to the width, not height. Indicates deficiency of blood, *yin*, or fluids.
Tight - an excess pulse, slightly wider than **wiry**. Often in superficial position. Indicates stagnation of blood, especially in trauma, or invasion of wind-cold.
Weak - the height of the pulse feels weak or soft. Indicates deficiency of *qi*.
Wide - the width of the pulse is wider than normal. Indicates excess of fluid, particularly damp or phlegm.
Wiry - a forceful, thin pulse. Indicates stagnation of *qi*, particularly liver *qi*.

QI (pronounced "chee")...The energy that flows through the acupuncture channels, and responsible for invigorating all organs, tissues and cells along its path. Also refers to the functional ability of individual organs, such as spleen *qi*, heart *qi*, lung *qi*, etc.

QI STAGNATION...*Qi* moves under healthy circumstances. When the *qi* stagnates, dysfunction and pain ensue. Can refer to either impaired circulation in the channels due to trauma, or congested energy in specific organs, particularly the stomach or liver. Stagnation of *qi* also includes accumulation of gas causing abdominal distension and belching.

SHEN ...Often translated as "spirit", *shen* includes the concepts of mind, consciousness, and higher spiritual connection . It is located in the heart. Disturbed *shen* manifests as insomnia, restlessness, muddled thinking, poor memory, uncomfortable dreaming, and manic disorders.

SPLEEN...includes the function of both spleen and pancreas, and is responsible for converting food to energy and blood, as well as regulating digestion.

SPLEEN-DAMP...In deficiencies of spleen *qi*, damp accumulates. This leads to water retention in the abdomen, loose or watery stools, and incomplete digestion; it is often the basis for phlegm congestion in the lungs.

SURFACE (Exterior)...The surface, rich in *wei qi*, is responsible for maintaining the body's internal homeostasis against a changeable environment. Exogenous invasions initially affect the surface, and the herbal approach is to dispel energetic invasions out through the skin, if the invasion has not proceeded too deeply into the body.

TOXIC HEAT...refers to exogenous toxic attacks (bacterial and viral) which can affect the body systemically with fever, attack specific organs, or affect the skin as inflamed boils.

WEI QI ...The most energetic aspect of *qi*, which circulates from the main channels to the exterior of the body. It is responsible for repulsing exogenous wind or toxic invasions, as well as contributing to the body's immune defense system.

WIND...Climatic disturbances in the air can induce pathogenic invasions if the *wei qi* is deficient. It attacks the surface of the body, further debilitates *wei qi*, and allows preponderance of toxic factors, causing the symptoms associated with flus and colds.

WIND-COLD...The body's response to a wind invasion exhibiting chills, nasal congestion, headache and body aches. Can occur as a response to over-exposure to wind and cold.

WIND-DAMP...In susceptible persons, exposure to wind in a damp environment or a pre-existing internal damp excess will cause rheumatism and joint pain. Accounts for various musculo-skeletal complaints.

WIND-HEAT...In wind invasions affecting people with pre-exisiting heat or deficiency-heat, colds are marked by fever, sore throat, and restlessness, or with the introduction of toxic viruses and bacteria.

WIND, INTERNAL...refers to an endogenous wind generated by liver fire. Symptoms include convulsions, muscle spasms, tics, severe headache, pressure behind eyes, or stroke. May follow a high fever.

WIND, LIVER...See Wind, Internal.

YANG ...The functional aspect of kidney *qi* which warms the body, and invigorates digestion, excretion, and sexual function. Deficiencies of *yang* allow the predominance of cold and hypofunction of the organs.

YIN ...The material and functional aspect of kidney *qi* which moistens and cools the liver, stomach, spleen, lungs, heart, throat, eyes and nose, and provides the basis for semen and vaginal fluids. Deficiencies of *yin* produce dryness and heat.

YING QI ...The *qi* that circulates in the acupuncture channels, and which nourishes the organs.

ZANG-FU...Taken together, *zang-fu* refers to organs (in distinction to acupuncture channels). The *zang* organs are considered to be more *yin* and solid (storing and slowly transforming) and include the heart, spleen-pancreas, lungs, kidneys and liver. The *fu* organs are considered more *yang* (functionally active) and hollow. They include the small and large intestines, gallbladder, stomach, and urinary bladder.

FORMULA NAMES BY PINYIN

An Zhong Tang	CARDAMON & FENNEL FORMULA
Ba Xian Chang Shou Wan	LONGEVITY FORMULA
Ba Zhen Tang	TANG KUEI & GINSENG EIGHT FORMULA
Ba Zheng Tang	DIANTHUS FORMULA
Ban Xia Hou Po Tang	PINELLIA & MAGNOLIA FORMULA
Bao He Tang	CITRUS & CRATAEGUS FORMULA
Bu Xue Tiao Jing Tang	BU TIAO FORMULA
Bu Zhong Yi Qi Tang	GINSENG & ASTRAGALUS FORMULA
Chai Hu Gui Zhi Tang	BUPLEURUM & CINNAMON FORMULA
Chai Hu Jia Long Gu Mu Li Tang	BUPLEURUM & DRAGON BONE FORMULA
Chuan Bi Tang	CHIANGHUO & TURMERIC FORMULA
Chuan Xin Lian Kang Yang Pian	ISATIS FORMULA
Chuan Xiong Cha Tiao Tang	CHUAN XIONG FORMULA
Dan Shen Yin	SALVIA PLUS FORMULA
Dan Zhi Xiao Yao San	BUPLEURUM & PEONY FORMULA
Dang Gui Shao Yao Tang	TANG KUEI & PEONY FORMULA
Ding Chuan Tang	MA HUANG & GINKGO PLUS FORMULA
Du Huo Ji Sheng Tang	DU HUO & LORANTHUS FORMULA
Er Chen Tang	CITRUS & PINELLIA FORMULA
Fang Feng Tong Sheng Tang	SILER & PLATYCODON FORMULA
Ge Gen Tang	PUERARIA FORMULA
Guan Jie Yam Wan	GUAN JIE FORMULA
Gui Pi Tang	GINSENG & LONGAN FORMULA
Gui Zhi Fu Ling Tang	CINNAMON & HOELEN FORMULA
Hong Hua Tao Ren Tang	CARTHAMUS & PERSICA FORMULA
Huang Lian Jie Du Tang	COPTIS & SCUTE FORMULA
Huang Qi Ling Zhi San	ASTRAGALUS & GANODERMA FORMULA
Jin Gu Die Shang Wan	JIN GU FORMULA
Jin Kui Shen Qi Jia Wan	REHMANNIA EIGHT PLUS FORMULA
Kang Ning Wan	CURING FORMULA
Li Dan Pai Shi Pian	LI DAN FORMULA
Liu Wei Di Huang Wan	REHMANNIA SIX FORMULA
Long Dan Xie Gan Tang	GENTIANA FORMULA

Qi Ju Di Huang Wan	LYCIUM & REHMANNIA FORMULA
Qing Bi Tang	PUERARIA "N" FORMULA
Qing Fei Tang	PLATYCODON & FRITILLARIA FORMULA
Qing Qi Hua Tan Tang Wan	PINELLIA "X" FORMULA
Qing Shang Juan Tong Tang	OPHIOPOGON & ASARUM FORMULA
Ren Shen Yang Rong Tang	GINSENG NUTRITIVE FORMULA
Sha Shen Mai Men Dong Tang	OPHIOPOGON PLUS FORMULA
Shen Ling Bai Zhu Tang	GINSENG & ATRACTYLODES FORMULA
Shou Wu Zhi	SHOU WU FORMULA
Shu Gan Wan	SHU KAN FORMULA
Shu Jing Huo Xue Tang	CLEMATIS & STEPHANIA FORMULA
Si Jun Zi Tang	FOUR GENTLEMEN FORMULA
Si Wu Tang	TANG KUEI FOUR FORMULA
Suan Zao Ren Tang	ZIZYPHUS FORMULA
Te Xiao Pai Shi Wan	PASSWAN FORMULA
Tian Ma Gou Teng Yin	GASTRODIA & UNCARIA FORMULA
Tian Wang Bu Xin Tang	GINSENG & ZIZYPHUS FORMULA
Tong Jing Wan	TO JING FORMULA
Wu Ling San	HOELEN FIVE FORMULA
Xiang Sha Liu Jun Zi Tang	SAUSSUREA & CARDAMON FORMULA
Xiao Chai Hu Tang	MINOR BUPLEURUM FORMULA
Xiao Feng San	TANG KUEI & ARCTIUM FORMULA
Xiao Qing Long Tang	MINOR BLUE DRAGON FORMULA
Xiao Yao San	BUPLEURUM & TANG KUEI FORMULA
Yi Yi Ren Tang	COIX FORMULA
Yin Chen Wu Ling Tang	CAPILLARIS & HOELEN FORMULA
Yin Qiao San	YIN QIAO FORMULA
Yu Ping Feng San	JADE SCREEN FORMULA
Zhi Bai Di Huang Wan	ANEM–PHELLO & REHMANNIA FORMULA
Zhong Gan Ling	ZHONG GAN LING FORMULA

HERBAL NAMING CROSS-REFERENCE

AH - astringent herbs (9)

CBH - clear blood heat (4)
CDH - clear damp-heat (4)
CIH - clear internal heat (4)
CS - calm *shen* (11)
CSH - clear summer-heat (4)
CTH - clear toxic heat (4)

DD - drain damp (diuretics) (6)
DWC - dispel wind-cold (spicy-warm herbs) (2)
DWD - expel wind-damp (6)
DWH - dispel wind-heat (spicy-cool herbs) (2)

EA - herbs for external application (15)
EP - expel parasites (14)

HC - harsh cathartics (diuretic purgatives) (13)

IB - invigorate blood (8)

OO - aromatic herbs to open orifices (senses) (10)

Pu purgatives (13)

RCA - relieve cough and asthma (3)
RFS - relieve food stagnation (7)
RSQ - regulate stagnant *qi* (7)

SB - stop bleeding (8)
SL - subdue liver *yang* and wind (12)

TB - tonify blood (8)
TPD - transform phlegm-damp (3)
TPH - transform phlegm-heat (3)
TQi - tonify *qi* (1)
TSD - fragrant herbs to transform spleen-damp (6)
TY -tonify *yang* (1)
TYi - tonify *yin* (1)

WI - warm the interior (dispel internal cold) (5)

1. **TONICS**
   TQi - tonify *qi*
   TBI - tonify blood
   TYa - tonify *yang*
   TYi - tonify *yin*

2. **Dispelling Exterior Conditions**
   DWC - dispel wind-cold (spicy-warm)
   DWH - dispel wind-heat (spicy-cool)

3. **HERBS TO TRANSFORM PHLEGM AND STOP COUGH**
   TPD - transform phlegm-damp
   TPH - transform phlegm-heat
   RCA - relieve cough and asthma

4. **HERBS TO CLEAR HEAT**
   CIH - clear internal heat
   CDH - clear damp-heat
   CBH - clear blood heat
   CTH - clear toxic heat
   CSH - clear summer-heat

5. **HERBS TO WARM THE INTERIOR AND DISPEL COLD**
   WI - warm the interior (dispel internal cold)

6. **HERBS TO DISPEL DAMP**
   DWD - dispel wind-damp
   TSD - fragrant herbs to transform spleen-damp
   DD - drain damp (diuretics)

7. **HERBS TO REGULATE** *QI*
   RSQ - regulate stagnant *qi*
   RFS - relieve food stagnation

8. **HERBS TO REGULATE BLOOD**
   SB - stop bleeding
   IB - invigorate blood

9. **ASTRINGENT HERBS**
   AH - astringent herbs

10. **AROMATIC HERBS TO OPEN ORIFICES**
    OO - aromatic herbs to open orifices (senses)

11. **HERBS TO CALM** *SHEN*
    CS - calm *shen*

12. **HERBS TO SUBDUE** *YANG* **AND EXTINGUISH WIND**
    SL - subdue liver *yang* and wind

13. **PURGATIVES**
    Pu - purgatives
    HC - harsh cathartics (diuretic purgatives)

14. **HERBS TO EXPEL PARASITES**
    EP - expel parasites

15. **HERBS FOR EXTERNAL APPLICATION**
    EA - herbs for external application

PHARMACEUTICAL-*PINYIN*	PART	DR. HSU-BRION	CATEGORY
Achyranthes *Niu Xi*	Radix	Achyranthes	TYi
Akebia *Mu Tong*	Caulis	Akebia	DD
Albizia *He Huan Pi*	Cortex	Albizia Bark	IB
Alisma *Ze Xie*	Rhizoma	Alisma	DD
Alpinia *Gao Liang Jiang*	Rhizoma		WI
Amomum *Bai Dou Kou*	Fructus		TSD
Amomum *Sha Ren*	Fructus	Cardamon	TSD
Andrographis *Chuan Xin Lian*	Herba		CTH
Anemarrhena *Zhi Mu*	Rhizoma	Anemarrhena	CIH
Angelica *Bai Zhi*	Radix	Angelica	DWC
Angelica *Dang Gui*	Radix	Tang–kuei	TBI
Angelica *Dang Gui Wei*	Radix		TBI
Angelica *Du Huo*	Radix	Tuhuo	DWD
Aquilaria *Chen Xiang*	Lignum	Aquilaria	RSQ
Arctium *Niu Bang Gen*	Radix		
Arctium *Niu Bang Zi*	Fructus	Arctium	DWH
Areca *Da Fu Pi*	Pericarpium	Areca	RSQ
Arisaema *Dan Nan Xing*	Rhizoma	Arisaema	TPD
Armeniaca *Xing Ren*	Semen	Apricot Seed	RCA
Artemesia *Ai Ye*	Folium	Artemesia	SB
Artemesia *Qing Hao*	Herba	Ching-hao	CSH
Artemesia *Yin Chen Hao*	Herba	Capillaris	DD
Asarum *Xi Xin*	Herba	Asarum	DWC
Asparagus *Tian Men Dong*	Radix	Asparagus	TYi
Astragalus *Huang Qi*	Radix	Astragalus	TQi
Atractylodes *Bai Zhu*	Rhizoma	White Atractylodes	TQi
Atractylodes *Cang Zhu*	Rhizoma	Atractylodes	TSD
Aurantium *Zhi Ke*	Fructus	Chih-ko	RSQ
Aurantium *Zhi Shi*	Fructus	Chih-shih	RSQ
Bambusa *Zhu Ru*	Caulis	Bamboo	TPH
Biota *Bai Zi Ren*	Semen	Biota	CS

AH: astringent herbs (9)
CBH: clear blood heat (4)
CDH: clear damp-heat (4)
CIH: clear internal heat (4)
CS: calm *shen* (11)
CSH: clear summer-heat (4)
CTH: clear toxic heat (4)
DD: drain damp (diuretics) (6)
DWC: dispel wind-cold (spicy-warm herbs) (2)
DWD: expel wind-damp (6)
DWH: dispel wind-heat (spicy-cool herbs) (2)

EA: for external application (15)
EP: expel parasites (14)
HC: harsh cathartics (diuretic purgatives) (13)
IB: invigorate blood (8)
OO: aromatic herbs to open orifices (senses) (10)
Pu: purgatives (13)
RCA: relieve cough and asthma (8)
RFS: relieve food stagnation (7)
RSQ: regulate stagnant *qi* (7)

SB: stop bleeding (8)
SL: subdue liver *yang* and wind (12)
TB: tonify blood (8)
TPD: transform phlegm-damp (3)
TPH: transform phlegm-heat (3)
TQI: tonify *qi* (1)
TSD: fragrant herbs to transform spleen-damp (6)
TYa: tonify *yang* (1)
TYi: tonify *yin* (1)
WI: warm the interior (dispel internal cold) (5)

PHARMACEUTICAL- *PINYIN*	PART	DR. HSU- BRION	CATEGORY
Bupleurum *Chai Hu*	Radix	Bupleurum	DWH
Capsella *Ji Cai*	Herba		CBH
Carthamus *Hong Hua*	Flos	Carthamus	IB
Caryophyllum *Ding Xiang*	Flos	Clove	WI
Cassia *Jue Ming Zi*	Semen	Cassia Seed	CIH
Chrysanthemum *Jua Hua*	Flos	Chrysanthemum	DWH
Cicada *Chan Tui*	Periostracum		DWH
Cimicifuga *Sheng Ma*	Rhizoma	Cimicifuga	DWH
Cinnamomum *Gui Zhi*	Ramulus	Cinnamon Twig	DWC
Cinnamomum *Rou Gui*	Cortex	Cinnamon Bark	WI
Cistanche *Rou Cong Rong*	Caulis	Cistanche	TYa
Citrus *Chen Pi*	Pericarpium	Citrus	RSQ
Citrus *Ju He*	Semen		RSQ
Citrus *Qing Pi*	Pericarpium	Blue Citrus	RSQ
Clematis *Wei Ling Xian*	Radix	Clematis	DWD
Codonopsis *Dang Shen*	Radix	Codonopsis	TQi
Coix *Yi Yi Ren*	Semen	Coix	DD
Coptis *Huang Lian*	Radix	Coptis	CDH
Cornus *Shan Zhu Yu*	Fructus	Cornus	AH
Corydalis *Yan Hu Suo*	Rhizoma	Corydalis	IB
Crataegus *Shan Zha*	Fructus	Crataegus	RFS
Curcuma *Jiang Huang*	Rhizoma		IB
Curcuma *Yu Jin*	Rhizoma	Curcuma	IB
Cuscuta *Tu Si Zi*	Semen	Cuscuta	TYa
Cyathula *Chuan Niu Xi*	Radix		IB
Cynomorium *Suo Yang*	Herba	Cynomorium	TYa
Cyperus *Xiang Fu*	Rhizoma	Cyperus	RSQ
Dendrobrium *Shi Hu*	Herba	Dendrobrium	TYi
Dianthus *Qu Mai*	Herba	Dianthus	DD
Dioscorea *Shan Yao*	Radix	Dioscorea	TQi

AH: astringent herbs (9)
CBH: clear blood heat (4)
CDH: clear damp-heat (4)
CIH: clear internal heat (4)
CS: calm *shen* (11)
CSH: clear summer-heat (4)
CTH: clear toxic heat (4)
DD: drain damp (diuretics) (6)
DWC: dispel wind-cold (spicy-warm herbs) (2)
DWD: expel wind-damp (6)
DWH: dispel wind-heat (spicy-cool herbs) (2)

EA: for external application (15)
EP: expel parasites (14)
HC: harsh cathartics (diuretic purgatives) (13)
IB: invigorate blood (8)
OO: aromatic herbs to open orifices (senses) (10)
Pu: purgatives (13)
RCA: relieve cough and asthma (3)
RFS: relieve food stagnation (7)
RSQ: regulate stagnant *qi* (7)

SB: stop bleeding (8)
SL: subdue liver *yang* and wind (12)
TB: tonify blood (8)
TPD: transform phlegm-damp (3)
TPH: transform phlegm-heat (3)
TQi: tonify *qi* (1)
TSD: fragrant herbs to transform spleen-damp (6)
TYa: tonify *yang* (1)
TYi: tonify *yin* (1)
WI: warm the interior (dispel internal cold) (5)

PHARMACEUTICAL- *PINYIN*	PART	DR. HSU- BRION	CATEGORY
Dipsacus *Xu Duan*	Radix	Dipsacus	TYa
Dolichoris *Bai Bian Dou*	Semen	Dolichos	CSH
Draconis *Long Gu*	Os	Dragon Bone	CS
Drynaria *Gu Sui Bu*	Rhizoma	Drynaria	TYa
Eleutheroginseng *Ci Wu Jia*	Radix	Eleutheroginseng	TQi
Ephedra *Ma Huang Gen*	Radix		AH
Ephedra *Ma Huang*	Herba	Ma-huang	DWC
Erythrinia *Hai Tong Pi*	Cortex		DWD
Eucommia *Du Zhong*	Cortex	Eucommia	TYa
Ficus *Wu Hua Guo Gen*	Radix		
Foeniculum *Hui Xiang*	Fructus	Fennel	WI
Forsythia *Lian Qiao*	Fructus	Forsythia	CTH
Fritillaria *Chuan Bei Ma*	Bulbus	Fritillaria	TPH
Ganoderma *Ling Zhi*	(Fungus)		TQi
Gardenia *Zhi Zi*	Fructus	Gardenia	CIH
Gastrodia *Tian Ma*	Rhizoma	Tian-ma	SL
Gelatinum *E Jiao*	Gelatinum		TBI
Gentiana *Long Dan Cao*	Radix	Gentiana	CDH
Gentiana *QIn Jiao*	Radix	Chin-chiu	DWD
Ginkgo *Yin Guo*	Fructus		AH
Ginseng *Ren Shen*	Radix	Ginseng	TQi
Glehnia *Bei Sha Shen*	Radix		TYi
Glycerrhiza *Gan Cao*	Radix	Licorice	TQi
Glycerrhiza *Zhi Gan Cao*	Radix	(Honey-fried Licorice)	TQi
Gypsum *Shi Gao*	Gypsum	Gypsum	CIH
Haliotis *Shi Jue Ming*	Concha	Haliotis	SL
Ilex *Mao Dong Qing*	Radix		CTH

AH: astringent herbs (9)
CBH: clear blood heat (4)
CDH: clear damp-heat (4)
CIH: clear internal heat (4)
CS: calm *shen* (11)
CSH: clear summer-heat (4)
CTH: clear toxic heat (4)
DD: drain damp (diuretics) (6)
DWC: dispel wind-cold (spicy-warm herbs) (2)
DWD: expel wind-damp (6)
DWH: dispel wind-heat (spicy-cool herbs) (2)

EA: for external application (15)
EP: expel parasites (14)
HC: harsh cathartics (diuretic purgatives) (13)
IB: invigorate blood (8)
OO: aromatic herbs to open orifices (senses) (10)
Pu: purgatives (13)
RCA: relieve cough and asthma (3)
RFS: relieve food stagnation (7)
RSQ: regulate stagnant *qi* (7)

SB: stop bleeding (8)
SL: subdue liver *yang* and wind (12)
TB: tonify blood (8)
TPD: transform phlegm-damp (3)
TPH: transform phlegm-heat (3)
TQi: tonify *qi* (1)
TSD: fragrant herbs to transform spleen-damp (6)
TYa: tonify *yang* (1)
TYi: tonify *yin* (1)
WI: warm the interior (dispel internal cold) (5)

PHARMACEUTICAL- *PINYIN*	PART	DR. HSU- BRION	CATEGORY
Inula *Xuan Fu Hua*	Flos	Inula	TPD
Isatis *Ban Lang Gen*	Radix	Isatis Root	CTH
Isatis *Da Qing Ye*	Herba	Isatis Leaf	CTH
Jujube *Da Zao*	Fructus	Jujube	TQi
Juncus *Deng Xin Cao*	Medula	Juncus	DD
Leonurus *Yi Mu Cao*	Herba	Leonurus	IB
Ligusticum *Chuan Xiong*	Rhizoma	Cnidium	IB
Ligustrum *Nu Zhen Zi*	Semen	Ligustrum	TYi
Lithosperm *Zi Cao*	Radix	Lithospermum	CBH
Litsea *Dou Chi Jing*	Radix		WI
Longan *Long Yan Rou*	Fructus	Longan	TBI
Lonicera *Jin Yin Hua*	Flos	Lonicera	CTH
Loranthus *Sang Ji Sheng*	Ramulus	Loranthus	TYi
Lycium *Gou Qi Zi*	Fructus	Lycium Fruit	TBI
Lygodium *Hai Jin Sha*	Spora	Lygodium	CTH
Lysimachia *Jin Qian Cao*	Herba		DD
Magnolia *Hou Po*	Cortex	Magnolia Bark	TSD
Magnolia *Xin Yi Hua*	Flos	Magnolia Flower	DWC
Massa Fermentata *Shen Chu*	Massa	Shen-chu	RFS
Mentha *Bo He*	Herba	Mentha	DWH
Millettia *Ji Xue Teng*	Radix	Millettia	IB
Mirabilite *Mang Xiao*	Natrium	Mirabilitum	Pu
Morinda *Ba Ji Tian*	Radix	Morinda	TYa
Morus *Sang Bai Pi*	Cortex	Morus Bark	RCA
Morus *Sang Shen*	Fructus	Morus Fruit	TBI
Morus *Sang Ye*	Herba	Morus Leaf	DWH
Moutan *Mu Dan Pi*	Cortex	Moutan	CBH
Myrrh *Mo Yao*	(Resin)	Myrrh	IB

AH: astringent herbs (9)
CBH: clear blood heat (4)
CDH: clear damp-heat (4)
CIH: clear internal heat (4)
CS: calm *shen* (11)
CSH: clear summer-heat (4)
CTH: clear toxic heat (4)
DD: drain damp (diuretics) (6)
DWC: dispel wind-cold (spicy-warm herbs) (2)
DWD: expel wind-damp (6)
DWH: dispel wind-heat (spicy-cool herbs) (2)

EA: for external application (15)
EP: expel parasites (14)
HC: harsh cathartics (diuretic purgatives) (13)
IB: invigorate blood (8)
OO: aromatic herbs to open orifices (senses) (10)
Pu: purgatives (13)
RCA: relieve cough and asthma (3)
RFS: relieve food stagnation (7)
RSQ: regulate stagnant *qi* (7)

SB: stop bleeding (8)
SL: subdue liver *yang* and wind (12)
TB: tonify blood (8)
TPD: transform phlegm-damp (3)
TPH: transform phlegm-heat (3)
TQi: tonify *qi* (1)
TSD: fragrant herbs to transform spleen-damp (6)
TYa: tonify *yang* (1)
TYi: tonify *yin* (1)
WI: warm the interior (dispel internal cold) (5)

PHARMACEUTICAL-PINYIN	PART	DR. HSU-BRION	CATEGORY
Nelumbo *Lian Zi*	Semen	Lotus Seed	AH
Notopterygium *Qiang Huo*	Rhizoma	Chiang-huo	DWC
Olibanum *Ru Xiang*	(Resin)	Frankincense	IB
Ophiopogon *Mai Men Dong*	Radix	Ophiopogon	TYi
Oryza *Gu Ya*	Fructus	(Sprouted Rice)	RFS
Ostrea *Mu Li*	Concha	Oyster Shell	CS
Paeonia *Bai Shao*	Radix	White Peonia	TBl
Paeonia *Chi Shao*	Radix	(Red) Peonia	IB
Perilla *Su Zi*	Semen	Perilla	RCA
Perilla *Zi Su Ye*	Folium	Perilla Leaf	DWC
Persica *Tao Ren*	Semen	Persica	IB
Phellodendron *Huang Bai*	Cortex	Phellodendron	CDH
Phragmites *Lu Gen*	Rhizoma	Phragmites	CIH
Pinellia *Ban Xia*	Rhizoma	Pinellia	TPD
Plantago *Che Qian Zi*	Semen	Plantago	DD
Platycodon *Jie Geng*	Radix	Platycodon	TPD
Pogostemon *Huo Xiang*	Herba	Agastache	TSD
Polygala *Yuan Zhi*	Radix	Polygala	CS
Polygonatum *Huang Jing*	Rhizoma		TQi
Polygonatum *Yu Zhu*	Rhizoma		TYi
Polygonum *Bian Xu*	Herba	Polygonum	DD
Polygonum *He Shou Wu*	Radix	Ho-sou-wu	TBl
Polygonum *Ye Jiao Teng*	Caulis	Polygonum Stem	CS
Polyporous *Zhu Ling*	(Fungus)	Polyporus	DD
Poria *Fu Ling*	(Fungus)	Hoelen	DD
Prunella *Xia Ku Cao*	Spica	Prunella	CIH
Pseudoginseng *Tian Qi*	Radix	Pseudoginseng	SB
Psoralea *Bu Gu Zhi*	Fructus	Psoralea	TYa
Pueraria *Ge Gen*	Radix	Pueraria	DWH

AH: astringent herbs (9)
CBH: clear blood heat (4)
CDH: clear damp-heat (4)
CIH: clear internal heat (4)
CS: calm *shen* (11)
CSH: clear summer-heat (4)
CTH: clear toxic heat (4)
DD: drain damp (diuretics) (6)
DWC: dispel wind-cold (spicy-warm herbs) (2)
DWD: expel wind-damp (6)
DWH: dispel wind-heat (spicy-cool herbs) (2)

EA: for external application (15)
EP: expel parasites (14)
HC: harsh cathartics (diuretic purgatives) (13)
IB: invigorate blood (8)
OO: aromatic herbs to open orifices (senses) (10)
Pu: purgatives (13)
RCA: relieve cough and asthma (3)
RFS: relieve food stagnation (7)
RSQ: regulate stagnant *qi* (7)

SB: stop bleeding (8)
SL: subdue liver *yang* and wind (12)
TB: tonify blood (8)
TPD: transform phlegm-damp (3)
TPH: transform phlegm-heat (3)
TQi: tonify *qi* (1)
TSD: fragrant herbs to transform spleen-damp (6)
TYa: tonify *yang* (1)
TYI: tonify *yin* (1)
WI: warm the interior (dispel internal cold) (5)

PHARMACEUTICAL-PINYIN	PART	DR. HSU-BRION	CATEGORY
Quinquefolium *Xi Yang Shen*	Radix	(American Ginseng)	TYi
Raphanus *Lai Fu Zi*	Semen	Raphanus	RFS
Rehmannia *Sheng Di Huang*	Radix	Rehmannia (fresh)	CBH
Rehmannia *Shu Di Huang*	Radix	Rehmannia (prepared)	TBI
Rheum *Da Huang*	Rhizoma	Rhubarb	Pu
Rosa *Jin Ying Zi*	Fructus	Rosa Fruit	AH
Salvia *Dan Shen*	Radix	Salvia	IB
Sanguis Draconis *Xue Jie*	(Resin)	(Dragon's Blood)	IB
Santalum *Tan Xiang*	Lignum	Santalum	RSQ
Saussurea *Mu Xiang*	Radix	Saussurea	RSQ
Schizandra *Wu Wei Zi*	Fructus	Schizandra	AH
Schizonepeta *Jing Jie*	Herba	Schizonepeta	DWC
Scrophularia *Xuan Shen*	Radix	Scrophularia	CBH
Scutellaria *Huang Qin*	Radix	Scute	CDH
Sesame *He Zhi Ma*	Semen	Sesame	TYi
Siler *Fang Feng*	Radix	Siler	DWC
Soja *Dan Dou Shi*	Semen	Soja	DWH
Sophora *Ku Shen*	Radix	Sophora	CDH
Sparganium *San Leng*	Rhizoma		IB
Stephania *Fang Ji*	Radix	Stephania	DD
Styrax *Su He Xiang*	(Resin)	Styrax	OO
Succinum *Hu Po*	(Resin)	Succinum (Amber)	CS
Talcum *Hua Shi*	Talcum	Talc	DD
Taraxacum *Pu Gong Ying*	Herba	Dandelion	CTH
Trichosanthes *Gua Lou Ren*	Semen	Trichosanthes Seed	TPH
Trichosanthes *Tian Hua Fen*	Radix	Trichosanthes Root	TPH
Tussilago *Kuan Dong Hua*	Flos	Tussilago	RCA

AH: astringent herbs (9)
CBH: clear blood heat (4)
CDH: clear damp-heat (4)
CIH: clear internal heat (4)
CS: calm *shen* (11)
CSH: clear summer-heat (4)
CTH: clear toxic heat (4)
DD: drain damp (diuretics) (6)
DWC: dispel wind-cold (spicy-warm herbs) (2)
DWD: expel wind-damp (6)
DWH: dispel wind-heat (spicy-cool herbs) (2)

EA: for external application (15)
EP: expel parasites (14)
HC: harsh cathartics (diuretic purgatives) (13)
IB: invigorate blood (8)
OO: aromatic herbs to open orifices (senses) (10)
Pu: purgatives (13)
RCA: relieve cough and asthma (3)
RFS: relieve food stagnation (7)
RSQ: regulate stagnant *qi* (7)

SB: stop bleeding (8)
SL: subdue liver *yang* and wind (12)
TB: tonify blood (8)
TPD: transform·phlegm-damp (3)
TPH: transform phlegm-heat (3)
TQI: tonify *qi* (1)
TSD: fragrant herbs to transform spleen-damp (6)
TYa: tonify *yang* (1)
TYI: tonify *yin* (1)
WI: warm the interior (dispel internal cold) (5)

PHARMACEUTICAL-PINYIN	PART	DR. HSU-BRION	CATEGORY
Uncaria *Gou Teng*	Ramulus	Gambir	SL
Verbena *Ma Bian Cao*	Herba		CTH
Viola *Zi Hua Di Ding*	Herba	Viola	CTH
Vitex *Man Jing Zi*	Fructus	Vitex	DWH
Zingiberis *Gan Jiang*	Rhizoma	Ginger (dried)	WI
Zingiberis *Sheng Jiang*	Rhizoma	Ginger (fresh)	DWC
Zizyphus *Suan Zao Ren*	Semen	Zizyphus	CS

AH: astringent herbs (9)
CBH: clear blood heat (4)
CDH: clear damp-heat (4)
CIH: clear internal heat (4)
CS: calm *shen* (11)
CSH: clear summer-heat (4)
CTH: clear toxic heat (4)
DD: drain damp (diuretics) (6)
DWC: dispel wind-cold (spicy-warm herbs) (2)
DWD: expel wind-damp (6)
DWH: dispel wind-heat (spicy-cool herbs) (2)

EA: for external application (15)
EP: expel parasites (14)
HC: harsh cathartics (diuretic purgatives) (13)
IB: invigorate blood (8)
OO: aromatic herbs to open orifices (senses) (10)
Pu: purgatives (13)
RCA: relieve cough and asthma (3)
RFS: relieve food stagnation (7)
RSQ: regulate stagnant *qi* (7)

SB: stop bleeding (8)
SL: subdue liver *yang* and wind (12)
TB: tonify blood (8)
TPD: transform phlegm-damp (3)
TPH: transform phlegm-heat (3)
TQi: tonify *qi* (1)
TSD: fragrant herbs to transform spleen-damp (6)
TYa: tonify *yang* (1)
TYi: tonify *yin* (1)
WI: warm the interior (dispel internal cold) (5)

INDEX OF FORMULAS
BY SYMPTOM AND APPLICATION

ABDOMINAL DISTENSION
Food stagnation
> CITRUS & CRATAEGUS FORMULA
> COIX FORMULA
> CURING FORMULA

Liver *qi* stagnation
> BUPLEURUM & CINNAMON FORMULA
> BUPLEURUM & TANG KUEI FORMULA

Liver *qi* stagnation with heat
> BUPLEURUM & PEONY FORMULA

Spleen *qi* deficiency
> GINSENG & ASTRAGALUS FORMULA
> SAUSSUREA & CARDAMON FORMULA

Stomach stagnation of *qi* and phlegm
> COIX FORMULA

ABDOMINAL PAIN
Liver *qi* stagnation
> BUPLEURUM & CINNAMON FORMULA

Stomach stagnation of *qi* and phlegm
> COIX FORMULA

Uterus blood stagnation
> CINNAMON & HOELEN FORMULA
> TO JING FORMULA

ABDOMINAL PAIN DURING PREGNANCY
TANG KUEI & PEONY FORMULA

ABSCESSES
ISATIS FORMULA

AMENORRHEA
Deficiency of blood
> SHOU WU FORMULA
> TANG KUEI FOUR FORMULA

Deficiency of *qi* and blood
> TANG KUEI & GINSENG EIGHT FORMULA

Uterus stagnation of blood
> CARTHAMUS & PERSICA FORMULA
> CINNAMON & HOELEN FORMULA
> TO JING FORMULA

(Amenorrhea continued)
Uterus stagnation of blood with blood deficiency
BU TIAO FORMULA

ANEMIA
Deficiency of blood
SHOU WU FORMULA
TANG KUEI FOUR FORMULA
Deficiency of *qi* and blood
GINSENG & LONGAN FORMULA
GINSENG NUTRITIVE FORMULA
TANG KUEI & GINSENG EIGHT FORMULA

ANXIETY AND NERVOUSNESS
BUPLEURUM & DRAGON BONE FORMULA
GINSENG & LONGAN FORMULA
GINSENG & ZIZYPHUS FORMULA
GINSENG NUTRITIVE FORMULA
MINOR BUPLEURUM FORMULA
ZIZYPHUS FORMULA

APPETITE, POOR
Deficiency of *qi*, blood and *yang*
GINSENG NUTRITIVE FORMULA
Liver *qi* stagnation
BUPLEURUM & TANG KUEI FORMULA
Liver *qi* stagnation with heat
BUPLEURUM & PEONY FORMULA
Liver *qi* stagnation with stomach *qi* stagnation
SHU KAN FORMULA
Liver *qi* stagnation with stomach phlegm and spleen *qi* deficiency
MINOR BUPLEURUM FORMULA
Stomach phlegm and damp
PINELLIA & MAGNOLIA FORMULA
Stomach phlegm-damp
CITRUS & PINELLIA FORMULA

ARTHRALGIA AND ARTHRITIS (Bi Syndromes)
Deficiency of blood
SHOU WU FORMULA
TANG KUEI FOUR FORMULA
Deficiency of kidney *qi*
DU HUO & LORANTHUS FORMULA
Deficiency of kidney *yang*
REHMANNIA EIGHT PLUS FORMULA
Deficiency of *qi*, blood, and *yang*
GINSENG & TANG KUEI TEN FORMULA

(Arthralgia and Arthritis (Bi Syndromes) continued)
Deficiency of *yin* with heat
ANEM-PHELLO & REHMANNIA FORMULA
Stagnation of liver *qi*
BUPLEURUM & CINNAMON FORMULA
MINOR BUPLEURUM FORMULA
Stagnation of *qi* and blood
CLEMATIS & STEPHANIA FORMULA
Stagnation of *qi* and blood due to trauma
JIN GU FORMULA
Wind–cold–damp
CHIANGHUO & TURMERIC FORMULA
CHUAN XIONG FORMULA
OPHIOPOGON & ASARUM FORMULA
Wind–cold–damp, damp dominent
HOELEN FIVE FORMULA
Wind–cold–damp, upper dominant
COIX FORMULA
Wind–cold–damp with stagnation of *qi* and blood
CLEMATIS & STEPHANIA FORMULA
Wind–damp–heat
GUAN JIE FORMULA

ASCITES
CAPILLARIS & HOELEN FORMULA
HOELEN FIVE FORMULA

ASCITES DUE TO JAUNDICE OR CIRRHOSIS
CAPILLARIS & HOELEN FORMULA

ASTHMA
MA HUANG & GINKGO PLUS FORMULA
MINOR BLUE DRAGON FORMULA
PINELLIA "X" FORMULA
PUERARIA FORMULA

BACK PAIN, LOWER
CHIANGHUO & TURMERIC FORMULA
CLEMATIS & STEPHANIA FORMULA
DU HUO & LORANTHUS FORMULA
REHMANNIA EIGHT PLUS FORMULA
TANG KUEI & PEONY FORMULA

BACK, WEAK
Kidney *yang* deficiency
REHMANNIA EIGHT PLUS FORMULA

(Back, Weak, kidney yang *deficiency continued)*
> DU HUO & LORANTHUS FORMULA

Kidney *yin* deficiency
> REHMANNIA SIX FORMULA

BELCHING
> CITRUS & CRATAEGUS FORMULA
> SHU KAN FORMULA

Bi **Syndromes (see ARTHRALGIA AND ARTHRITIS)**

BLADDER STONE
> DIANTHUS FORMULA

BLOOD CHOLESTEROL AND LIPIDS, HIGH
> CITRUS & CRATAEGUS FORMULA
> SALVIA PLUS FORMULA
> SHOU WU FORMULA

BLURRY VISION
> BUPLEURUM & TANG KUEI FORMULA
> LYCIUM & REHMANNIA FORMULA

BREAST DISTENSION
> BUPLEURUM & PEONY FORMULA
> BUPLEURUM & TANG KUEI FORMULA

BREATHING, DIFFICULT
> LONGEVITY FORMULA
> MA HUANG & GINKGO PLUS FORMULA
> MINOR BLUE DRAGON FORMULA

Bronchitis (see COUGH)

CATARACTS
> LYCIUM & REHMANNIA FORMULA

CERVICAL DISORDERS
> PUERARIA FORMULA

CHEST CONSTRICTION
> MA HUANG & GINKGO PLUS FORMULA
> PINELLIA "X" FORMULA
> SALVIA PLUS FORMULA

CHILLS AND FEVERS, ALTERNATING
> MINOR BUPLEURUM FORMULA

CHRONIC FATIGUE SYNDROME
Toxic virus
ISATIS FORMULA
Deficiency of *qi* and *yin*
ASTRAGALUS & GANODERMA FORMULA
Deficiency of *yin* with heat
ANEM-PHELLO & REHMANNIA FORMULA

COMMON COLD
Alternating chills and fever
MINOR BUPLEURUM FORMULA
Runny nose
MINOR BLUE DRAGON FORMULA
Stiff neck and headache
PUERARIA FORMULA
Viral infection
ISATIS FORMULA
ZHONG GAN LING FORMULA
Wind-heat invasion, early stage
YIN QIAO FORMULA

CONSTIPATION
Deficiency of *yin*
OPHIOPOGON PLUS FORMULA
REHMANNIA SIX FORMULA
Premenstrual
BUPLUEURUM & TANG KUEI FORMULA
With fever
SILER & PLATYCODON FORMULA

COSTAL DISTENSION WITH PAIN
SHU KAN FORMULA

COUGH
Lung phlegm–damp
CITRUS & PINELLIA FORMULA
MINOR BLUE DRAGON FORMULA
PINELLIA & MAGNOLIA FORMULA
Lung phlegm-heat
PINELLIA "X" FORMULA
Lung phlegm-heat with yin deficiency
PLATYCODON & FRITILLARIA FORMULA
Lung *qi* deficiency with slight phlegm
MA HUANG & GINKGO PLUS FORMULA
Lung *yin* deficiency (dry cough)
LONGEVITY FORMULA

(Cough, lung yin *deficiency (dry cough) continued)*
OPHIOPOGON PLUS FORMULA
Smoker's cough
PLATYCODON & FRITILLARIA FORMULA

DEPRESSION
BUPLEURUM & TANG KUEI FORMULA

DIARRHEA OR LOOSE STOOLS
Accumulation of damp
HOELEN FIVE FORMULA
Damp-heat
CAPILLARIS & HOELEN FORMULA
Spleen *qi* deficiency
GINSENG & ASTRAGALUS FORMULA
SAUSSUREA & CARDAMON FORMULA
Stomach phlegm
CITRUS & PINELLIA FORMULA

DIGESTION, POOR
Deficiency of *qi* and blood
GINSENG & LONGAN FORMULA
TANG KUEI & GINSENG EIGHT FORMULA
Liver *qi* stagnation with stomach *qi* stagnation
SHU KAN FORMULA
Spleen *qi* deficiency
GINSENG & ASTRAGALUS FORMULA
SAUSSUREA & CARDAMON FORMULA
Spleen *qi* deficiency with accumulation of cold and damp
HOELEN FIVE FORMULA

DIZZINESS
Deficiency of blood
SHOU WU FORMULA
TANG KUEI FOUR FORMULA
Deficiency of *qi* and blood
GINSENG & LONGAN FORMULA
TANG KUEI & GINSENG EIGHT FORMULA
Heart blood and *yin* deficiency
ZIZYPHUS FORMULA
Heart *yin* deficiency
GINSENG & ZIZYPHUS FORMULA
Liver *qi* stagnation
BUPLEURUM & TANG KUEI FORMULA
Liver *qi* stagnation with heat
BUPLEURUM & PEONY FORMULA

(Dizziness continued)

Liver *yin* deficiency
>> LYCIUM & REHMANNIA FORMULA
>> REHMANNIA SIX FORMULA

Liver *yin* deficiency with liver *yang* rising
>> GASTRODIA & UNCARIA FORMULA

Stomach phlegm
>> CITRUS & PINELLIA FORMULA

DYSMENORRHEA

> BU TIAO FORMULA
> CARTHAMUS & PERSICA FORMULA
> CINNAMON & HOELEN FORMULA
> TO JING FORMULA

EARACHES

> PUERARIA "N" FORMULA

EAR–RINGING

> GASTRODIA & UNCARIA FORMULA

ECZEMA

> TANG KUEI & ARCTIUM FORMULA

EDEMA

> CAPILLARIS & HOELEN FORMULA

EDEMA IN LIMBS

> CLEMATIS & STEPHANIA FORMULA
> COIX FORMULA
> HOELEN FIVE FORMULA

EMPHYSEMA

> MA HUANG & GINKGO PLUS FORMULA
> MINOR BLUE DRAGON FORMULA
> PINELLIA "X" FORMULA
> PLATYCODON & FRITILLARIA FORMULA

ENDOMETRIOSIS

> CINNAMON & HOELEN FORMULA

EPIGASTRIC DISTENSION

Food stagnation
>> CITRUS & CRATAEGUS FORMULA
>> CURING FORMULA

(*Epigastric Distension continued*)
    Liver *qi* stagnation affecting stomach
        SHU KAN FORMULA
    Liver *qi* stagnation with spleen *qi* deficiency
        MINOR BUPLEURUM FORMULA
    Stomach phlegm
        CITRUS & PINELLIA FORMULA
    Stomach hyperacidity (ulcer)
        CARDAMON & FENNEL FORMULA
    Stomach phlegm and damp
        PINELLIA & MAGNOLIA FORMULA

EPIGASTRIC PAIN
    Food stagnation
        CITRUS & CRATAEGUS FORMULA
        CURING FORMULA
    Liver *qi* stagnation
        BUPLEURUM & CINNAMON FORMULA
        BUPLEURUM & TANG KUEI FORMULA
    Liver *qi* stagnation affecting stomach
        SHU KAN FORMULA
    Stomach blood stagnation (ulcer)
        CARDAMON & FENNEL FORMULA
    Stomach hyperacidity
        CARDAMON & FENNEL FORMULA

EPILEPSY
    BUPLEURUM & DRAGON BONE FORMULA

EPSTEIN–BARR VIRUS
    ISATIS FORMULA

EYE PRESSURE
    GASTRODIA & UNCARIA FORMULA
    GENTIANA FORMULA

EYE, RED
    BUPLEURUM & PEONY FORMULA
    GENTIANA FORMULA

EYE, SPOTS IN VISION
    Liver blood deficiency
        SHOU WU FORMULA
        TANG KUEI & GINSENG EIGHT FORMULA
    Liver *yin* deficiency
        LYCIUM & CHRYSANTHEMUM FORMULA

EYES, DRY
> GASTRODIA & UNCARIA FORMULA
> LYCIUM & REHMANNIA FORMULA
> REHMANNIA SIX FORMULA

EYESIGHT (see Vision)

FATIGUE
> Deficiency of blood
>> SHOU WU FORMULA
>> TANG KUEI FOUR FORMULA
> Deficiency of lung *yin*
>> OPHIOPOGON PLUS FORMULA
> Deficiency of *qi* and blood
>> GINSENG & LONGAN FORMULA
>> TANG KUEI & GINSENG EIGHT FORMULA
> Deficiency of *qi* and *yin*
>> ASTRAGALUS & GANODERMA FORMULA
> Deficiency of *qi*, blood and *yang*
>> GINSENG NUTRITIVE FORMULA
> Following prolonged illness
>> TANG KUEI & GINSENG EIGHT FORMULA
>> GINSENG NUTRITIVE FORMULA
> Kidney *yin* deficiency
>> REHMANNIA SIX FORMULA
> Menstrual, due to deficiency of *qi* and *yang*
>> BU TIAO FORMULA
> Post-partum or post-surgery
>> GINSENG NUTRITIVE FORMULA
> Spleen *qi* deficiency
>> GINSENG & ASTRAGALUS FORMULA
>> SAUSSUREA & CARDAMON FORMULA

FEVER
> Afternoon low grade (deficiency of *yin* with heat)
>> ANEM-PHELLO & REHMANNIA FORMULA
>> LONGEVITY FORMULA
> High fever during common cold
>> SILER & PLATYCODON FORMULA
>> ZHONG GAN LING FORMULA

FLATULENCE
> Food stagnation
>> CITRUS & CRATAEGUS FORMULA
>> CURING FORMULA
> Liver *qi* stagnation
>> BUPLEURUM & CINNAMON FORMULA

(Flatulence continued)
> Liver *qi* stagnation affecting stomach
>> SHU KAN FORMULA
> Spleen *qi* deficiency
>> GINSENG & ASTRAGALUS FORMULA
>> SAUSSUREA & CARDAMON FORMULA

FLU
> ISATIS FORMULA
> MINOR BUPLEURUM FORMULA
> SILER & PLATYCODON FORMULA
> YIN QIAO FORMULA
> ZHONG GAN LING FORMULA

FOOD ALLERGIES
> BUPLEURUM & PEONY FORMULA
> BUPLEURUM & TANG KUEI FORMULA
> MINOR BUPLEURUM FORMULA

FOOD POISONING
> CURING FORMULA
> PINELLIA & MAGNOLIA FORMULA

FOOD STAGNATION
> CITRUS & CRATAEGUS FORMULA
> CURING FORMULA
> PINELLIA & MAGNOLIA FORMULA
> SAUSSUREA & CARDAMON FORMULA

GALLBLADDER INFLAMMATION
> GENTIANA FORMULA
> LI DAN FORMULA

GALLSTONES
> GENTIANA FORMULA
> LI DAN FORMULA

GLAUCOMA
> LYCIUM & REHMANNIA FORMULA

GLOBUS HYSTERICUS
> PINELLIA & MAGNOLIA FORMULA

GOITER
> CITRUS & PINELLIA FORMULA

HABITUAL MISCARRIAGE
  TANG KUEI & PEONY FORMULA

HAIR, DRY OR BRITTLE
  SHOU WU FORMULA
  TANG KUEI & GINSENG EIGHT FORMULA
  TANG KUEI FOUR FORMULA

HANGOVER
  CITRUS & CRATAEGUS FORMULA
  CITRUS & PINELLIA FORMULA
  CURING FORMULA

HEADACHE
  Common cold
    OPHIOPOGON & ASARUM FORMULA
    PUERARIA FORMULA
  Liver and stomach dysharmony
    BUPLEURUM & CINNAMON FORMULA
  Liver or gallbladder fire
    GENTIANA FORMULA
  Liver *qi* stagnation
    BUPLEURUM & TANG KUEI FORMULA
    MINOR BUPLEURUM FORMULA
  Liver *qi* stagnation with heat
    BUPLEURUM & PEONY FORMULA
  Liver *qi* stagnation with rising liver *yang*
    BUPLEURUM & DRAGON BONE FORMULA
  Liver *qi* stagnation with stagnation in the channels
    OPHIOPOGON & ASARUM FORMULA
  Liver *yin* deficiency with rising liver *yang*
    GASTRODIA & UNCARIA FORMULA
  Viral encephaly
    CAPILLARIS & HOELEN FORMULA
    HOELEN FIVE FORMULA
    ISATIS FORMULA

HEMATURIA
  CAPILLARIS & HOELEN FORMULA

HEPATITIS
  Acute
    GENTIANA FORMULA
    ISATIS FORMULA
    LI DAN FORMULA

(Hepatitis continued)
Chronic
CAPILLARIS AND HOELEN FORMULA
LI DAN FORMULA
MINOR BUPLEURUM FORMULA

HEPATOMEGALY
CARTHAMUS & PERSICA FORMULA
ISATIS FORMULA
SALVIA PLUS FORMULA

HERNIA
GINSENG & ASTRAGALUS FORMULA

HERPES (oral or genital)
GENTIANA FORMULA
ISATIS FORMULA

HICCUP
SHU KAN FORMULA

HIVES
TANG KUEI & ARCTIUM FORMULA

HOT FLASHING (MENOPAUSE)
ANEM-PHELLO & REHMANNIA FORMULA
BUPLEURUM & PEONY FORMULA

HOT PALMS AND SOLES
ANEM-PHELLO & REHMANNIA FORMULA

HYPERACTIVE THYROID
GINSENG & ZIZYPHUS FORMULA

HYPERTENSION
BUPLEURUM & DRAGON BONE FORMULA
GASTRODIA & UNCARIA FORMULA
LYCIUM & REHMANNIA FORMULA

HYPOGLYCEMIA
GINSENG & ASTRAGALUS FORMULA
MINOR BUPLEURUM FORMULA
SHU KAN FORMULA

INCREASING RESISTANCE TO DISEASE
JADE SCREEN FORMULA

INFERTILITY
Blood stagnation
  CARTHAMUS & PERSICA FORMULA
Deficiency of *qi* and blood
  TANG KUEI & PEONY FORMULA
Liver *qi* stagnation
  BUPLEURUM & TANG KUEI FORMULA
Liver *qi* stagnation with heat
  BUPLEURUM & PEONY FORMULA
Uterus blood stagnation with deficiency of *qi* and *yang*
  BU TIAO FORMULA
Uterus blood stagnation with deficiency of *yang*
  CINNAMON & HOELEN FORMULA

Injury (see TRAUMATIC INJURY)

INSOMNIA
Deficiency of blood
  SHOU WU FORMULA
  TANG KUEI FOUR FORMULA
Deficiency of *qi* and *yin*
  ASTRAGALUS & GANODERMA FORMULA
Deficiency of *qi*, blood, and *yang*
  GINSENG NUTRITIVE FORMULA
Deficiency of *yin* with heat
  ANEM-PHELLO & REHMANNIA FORMULA
Heart blood and *yin* deficiency
  ZIZYPHUS FORMULA
Heart blood deficiency with spleen *qi* deficiency
  GINSENG & LONGAN FORMULA
  GINSENG NUTRITIVE FORMULA
Heart *yin* deficiency
  GINSENG & ZIZYPHUS FORMULA
Liver *qi* stagnation with rising liver *yang*
  BUPLEURUM & DRAGON BONE FORMULA
Liver *qi* stagnation with spleen *qi* deficiency
  MINOR BUPLEURUM FORMULA
Wind-heat invasion (common cold)
  YIN QIAO FORMULA

Irregular Menses (see MENSES, IRREGULAR)

Irregular Pulse (see PULSE, IRREGULAR)

IRRITABILITY
Liver *qi* stagnation
  BUPLEURUM & TANG KUEI FORMULA

(Irritability continued)
> Liver *qi* stagnation with heat
> > BUPLEURUM & PEONY FORMULA
> Liver *qi* stagnation with rising liver *yang*
> > BUPLEURUM & DRAGON BONE FORMULA
> Liver *qi* stagnation with spleen *qi* deficency
> > BUPLEURUM & CINNAMON FORMULA

JAUNDICE (also see HEPATITIS)
> CAPILLARIS & HOELEN FORMULA

JOINTS AND LIMBS, PAINFUL (LOWER)
> CLEMATIS & STEPHANIA FORMULA

JOINTS AND LIMBS, PAINFUL (UPPER)
> CHIANGHUO & TURMERIC FORMULA
> COIX FORMULA

KIDNEY INFECTION
> ANEM-PHELLO & REHMANNIA FORMULA
> DIANTHUS FORMULA

KIDNEY STONE
> DIANTHUS FORMULA
> PASSWAN FORMULA

KNEES, COLD OR WEAK
> REHMANNIA EIGHT PLUS FORMULA

LEUKORRHEA
> Deficiency of spleen *qi*
> > GINSENG & ATRACTYLODES FORMULA
> Liver damp-heat
> > GENTIANA FORMULA
> Uterus blood stagnation
> > CINNAMON & HOELEN FORMULA

LIMBS, ACHING
> TANG KUEI & GINSENG EIGHT FORMULA

LIMBS, COLD
> REHMANNIA EIGHT PLUS FORMULA

Liver, Swollen (see HEPATOMEGALY)

Low Back Pain (see BACK PAIN, LOWER)

Lower Back, Weak (see BACK, WEAK)

LYMPH GLANDS, SWOLLEN
ISATIS FORMULA

MANIA
BUPLEURUM & DRAGON BONE FORMULA

MASTITIS
ISATIS FORMULA

MEASLES
ISATIS FORMULA
YIN QIAO FORMULA

MEMORY, POOR
GINSENG & LONGAN FORMULA

MENOPAUSAL HOT FLASHING
ANEM-PHELLO & REHMANNIA FORMULA
BUPLEURUM & PEONY FORMULA

MENSES, DELAYED
Deficiency of blood
SHOU WU FORMULA
TANG KUEI FOUR FORMULA
Deficiency of *qi* and blood
TANG KUEI & GINSENG EIGHT FORMULA

MENSES, IRREGULAR
Deficiency of blood
SHOU WU FORMULA
TANG KUEI FOUR FORMULA
Deficiency of *qi* and blood
TANG KUEI & GINSENG EIGHT FORMULA
Liver *qi* stagnation
BUPLEURUM & TANG KUEI FORMULA
Liver *qi* stagnation with heat
BUPLEURUM & PEONY FORMULA
Liver *yin* deficiency
LYCIUM & REHMANNIA FORMULA
Uterus blood stagnation
CARTHAMUS & PERSICA FORMULA
CINNAMON & HOELEN FORMULA
Uterus blood stagnation with deficiency of *qi* and *yang*
BU TIAO FORMULA

MENSTRUAL CLOTS
CARTHAMUS & PERSICA FORMULA
TO JING FORMULA

Menstrual Cramps (see DYSMENORRHEA)

Menstrual Pain (see DYSMENORRHEA)

Migraine (see HEADACHES)

MORNING SICKNESS
CURING FORMULA
PINELLIA & MAGNOLIA FORMULA
SAUSSUREA & CARDAMON FORMULA

MOTION SICKNESS
CURING FORMULA

MOUTH, DRY
REHMANNIA SIX FORMULA

MOVEMENT OF JOINTS AND LIMBS, DIFFICULT
CHIANGHUO & TURMERIC FORMULA
CLEMATIS & STEPHANIA FORMULA
COIX FORMULA

MUMPS
ISATIS FORMULA

MUSCULAR TENSION
BUPLEURUM & CINNAMON FORMULA
BUPLEURUM & DRAGON BONE FORMULA
BUPLEURUM & TANG KUEI FORMULA
MINOR BUPLEURUM FORMULA

NAILS, POOR
TANG KUEI & GINSENG EIGHT FORMULA

NASAL CONGESTION
MINOR BLUE DRAGON FORMULA
PUERARIA "N" FORMULA

NAUSEA
Deficiency of spleen *qi*
SAUSSUREA & CARDAMON FORMULA
Dysharmony of liver and stomach
BUPLEURUM & CINNAMON FORMULA

(Nausea continued)
Stomach phlegm
> CITRUS & PINELLIA FORMULA

Stomach phlegm and damp
> PINELLIA & MAGNOLIA FORMULA

Stomach *qi* stagnation with phlegm
> CURING FORMULA

NECK AND SHOULDER TENSION
OPHIOPOGON & ASARUM FORMULA
PUERARIA FORMULA

Nervousness, (see ANXIETY AND NERVOUSNESS)

NIGHT SWEATS
ANEM-PHELLO & REHMANNIA FORMULA
ZIZYPHUS FORMULA

OVARIAN CYST
CARTHAMUS & PERSICA FORMULA
TO JING FORMULA

Painful Urination (see URINARY DISTURBANCE)

PALPITATION
Deficiency of blood
> SHOU WU FORMULA
> TANG KUEI FOUR FORMULA

Deficiency of *qi*, blood, and *yang*
> GINSENG NUTRITIVE FORMULA

Heart blood and *yin* deficiency
> ZIZYPHUS FORMULA

Heart blood deficiency with spleen *qi* deficiency
> GINSENG & LONGAN FORMULA
> GINSENG NUTRITIVE FORMULA

Heart *yin* deficiency
> GINSENG & ZIZYPHUS FORMULA

Liver *qi* stagnation with liver *yang* rising
> BUPLEURUM & DRAGON BONE FORMULA

PELVIC INFLAMATORY DISEASE
DIANTHUS FORMULA
GENTIANA FORMULA

PLACENTA, RETAINED
CINNAMON & HOELEN FORMULA

PLUM–PIT SENSATION IN THROAT
PINELLIA & MAGNOLIA FORMULA

PNEUMONIA
PINELLIA "X" FORMULA

Poor Appetite (see APPETITE, POOR)

Poor Digestion (see DIGESTION, POOR)

POST-MENSTRUAL FATIGUE
Deficiency of blood
SHOU WU FORMULA
TANG KUEI FOUR FORMULA
Deficiency of *qi* and blood
TANG KUEI & GINSENG EIGHT FORMULA
Liver *yin* deficiency
LYCIUM & REHMANNIA FORMULA

POST-PARTUM FATIGUE
ASTRAGALUS & GANODERMA FORMULA
GINSENG NUTRITIVE FORMULA
SHOU WU FORMULA
TANG KUEI & GINSENG EIGHT FORMULA
TANG KUEI & PEONY FORMULA
TANG KUEI FOUR FORMULA

POST–SURGERY FATIGUE
ASTRAGALUS & GANODERMA FORMULA
GINSENG NUTRITIVE FORMULA

PREMATURE EJACULATIONS
Deficiency of *yin*
ANEM-PHELLO & REHMANNIA FORMULA
Deficiency of *yang*
REHMANNIA EIGHT PLUS FORMULA

PREMENSTRUAL SYNDROME (PMS)
Liver *qi* stagnation
BUPLEURUM & TANG KUEI FORMULA
Liver *qi* stagnation with heat
BUPLEURUM & PEONY FORMULA
Liver *yin* deficiency (combine with above)
LYCIUM & REHMANNIA FORMULA

PREMENSTRUAL WATER RETENTION
TANG KUEI & PEONY FORMULA

PROLAPSE OF INTESTINE, RECTUM OR UTERUS
GINSENG & ASTRAGALUS FORMULA

PROSTATITIS, ACUTE
DIANTHUS FORMULA
GENTIANA FORMULA

PROSTATITIS, CHRONIC
GINSENG & ASTRAGALUS FORMULA

PULSE, IRREGULAR
GINSENG & ZIZYPHUS FORMULA
GINSENG NUTRITIVE FORMULA

RASH
TANG KUEI & ARCTIUM FORMULA

RED EYE
BUPLEURUM & PEONY FORMULA
GENTIANA FORMULA

RESTLESSNESS
Liver *qi* stagnation
MINOR BUPLEURUM FORMULA
Liver *qi* stagnation with heat
BUPLEURUM & PEONY FORMULA
Liver *qi* stagnation with rising liver *yang*
BUPLEURUM & DRAGON BONE FORMULA
Heart *yin* deficiency
GINSENG & ZIZYPHUS FORMULA

RHEUMATISM (see Arthritis and Arthralgia)

RHEUMATOID ARTHRITIS
CLEMATIS & STEPHANIA FORMULA
GUAN JIE FORMULA

RHINITIS
PUERARIA "N" FORMULA
MINOR BLUE DRAGON FORMULA

RUNNY NOSE
MINOR BLUE DRAGON FORMULA

SCIATICA
CLEMATIS & STEPHANIA FORMULA

SCROTAL ECZEMA
GENTIANA FORMULA

SCROTAL HYDROCELE
CAPILLARIS & HOELEN FORMULA
HOELEN FIVE FORMULA

SEXUAL EXHAUSTION, MALE
GINSENG NUTRITIVE FORMULA
SHOU WU FORMULA

SHOULDERS AND NECK, ACHING
Liver *qi* stagnation
MINOR BUPLEURUM FORMULA
Wind-cold invasion (common cold)
PUERARIA FORMULA
Wind-heat invasion (common cold)
YIN QIAO FORMULA

SINUS CONGESTION
MINOR BLUE DRAGON FORMULA
OPHIOPOGON & ASARUM FORMULA
PUERARIA "N" FORMULA
YIN QIAO FORMULA

SINUS HEADACHE
OPHIOPOGON & ASARUM FORMULA
PUERARIA "N" FORMULA

SINUS PHLEGM
PINELLIA "X" FORMULA

SKIN DISORDERS
TANG KUEI & ARCTIUM FORMULA

SKIN, DRY
SHOU WU FORMULA
TANG KUEI & GINSENG EIGHT FORMULA

Sleep, Restless (see INSOMNIA)

SMOKING AND DRUG WITHDRAWAL
BUPLEURUM & DRAGON BONE FORMULA
MINOR BUPLEURUM FORMULA

SNORING
PUERARIA "N" FORMULA

SPASMS
>   CHIANGHUO & TURMERIC FORMULA

SPERMATORRHEA
>   ANEM-PHELLO & REHMANNIA FORMULA

SPOTS IN VISION
>   TANG KUEI & GINSENG EIGHT FORMULA

STOMACH FLU
>   CURING FORMULA

Stomach Pain (see EPIGASTRIC PAIN)

STOOLS, DRY
>   REHMANNIA SIX FORMULA

STOOLS, ERRATIC (diarrhea, loose, pasty, or constipation)
>   CITRUS & CRATAEGUS FORMULA
>   CURING FORMULA
>   GINSENG & ASTRAGALUS FORMULA
>   SAUSSUREA & CARDAMON FORMULA

STOOLS, LOOSE
>   GINSENG & ASTRAGALUS FORMULA
>   REHMANNIA EIGHT PLUS FORMULA
>   SAUSSUREA & CARDAMON FORMULA
>   TANG KUEI & GINSENG EIGHT FORMULA

STREPT THROAT
>   COPTIS & SCUTE FORMULA
>   ISATIS FORMULA
>   ZHONG GAN LING FORMULA

STROKE
>   GASTRODIA & UNCARIA FORMULA

SWOLLEN LIVER (HEPATOMEGALY)
>   CARTHAMUS & PERSICA FORMULA

TACHYCARDIA
>   ZIZYPHUS FORMULA

TEMPORAL–MANDIBULAR JOINT PAIN (TMJ)
>   OPHIOPOGON & ASARUM FORMULA

TESTICLES SWOLLEN
GENTIANA FORMULA

Thick Nasal Discharge (see SINUS CONGESTION)

THIRST
ANEM-PHELLO & REHMANNIA FORMULA
LONGEVITY FORMULA
OPHIOPOGON PLUS FORMULA
REHMANNIA SIX FORMULA

THROAT, SORE
ISATIS FORMULA
YIN QIAO FORMULA

TIDAL FEVERS
ANEM-PHELLO & REHMANNIA FORMULA
ASTRAGALUS & GANODERMA FORMULA

TONSILLITIS
YIN QIAO FORMULA

TRAUMATIC INJURY
CARTHAMUS & PERSICA FORMULA
JIN GU FORMULA

TRIGEMINAL NEURALGIA
OPHIOPOGON & ASARUM FORMULA

ULCER, STOMACH
CARDAMON & FENNEL FORMULA
GINSENG & LONGAN FORMULA

URINARY DISTURBANCE
CAPILLARIS & HOELEN FORMULA
DIANTHUS FORMULA
GENTIANA FORMULA
HOELEN FIVE FORMULA

URINARY FREQUENCY
REHMANNIA EIGHT PLUS FORMULA

URINARY RETENTION
HOELEN FIVE FORMULA
REHMANNIA EIGHT PLUS FORMULA

URINARY TRACT INFECTION
    ANEM-PHELLO & REHMANNIA FORMULA
    DIANTHUS FORMULA
    GENTIANA FORMULA

URINE, CONCENTRATED OR PAINFUL
    GENTIANA FORMULA

UTERINE BLEEDING
Deficiency of blood
    SHOU WU FORMULA
    TANG KUEI FOUR FORMULA
Deficiency of *qi* and blood
    GINSENG & LONGAN FORMULA
    TANG KUEI & GINSENG EIGHT FORMULA
Deficiency of *yin* with heat
    ANEM-PHELLO & REHMANNIA FORMULA
Spleen *qi* deficiency
    GINSENG & ASTRAGALUS FORMULA
Uterus blood stagnation with deficiency of *qi* and *yang*
    BU TIAO FORMULA

UTERINE FIBROIDS
    CARTHAMUS & PERSICA FORMULA
    CINNAMON & HOELEN FORMULA
    TO JING FORMULA

VAGINITIS
    GENTIANA FORMULA

VERTEBRAL SUBLUXATIONS
    BUPLEURUM & CINNAMON FORMULA

Vertigo (see DIZZINESS)

VIRAL INFECTIONS
    ISATIS FORMULA

VISION, BLURRY OR WEAK
Liver blood deficiency
    SHOU WU FORMULA
Liver *yin* deficiency
    LYCIUM & CHRYSANTHEMUM FORMULA

VOMITING
    BUPLEURUM & CINNAMON FORMULA

(Vomiting continued)
      CITRUS & PINELLIA FORMULA
      PINELLIA & MAGNOLIA FORMULA

VOMITING OF BLOOD
      CARDAMON & FENNEL FORMULA

WATER RETENTION
      HOELEN FIVE FORMULA
      TANG KUEI & PEONY FORMULA

WATERY PHLEGM IN MOUTH
      CITRUS & PINELLIA FORMULA

***WEI QI* (DEFENSIVE ENERGY) WEAK**
      ASTRAGALUS & GANODERMA FORMULA
      JADE SCREEN FORMULA

SUPPLIERS OF PRODUCTS

ZAND Chinese Classics,
Liquid herbal extracts:
McZand Herbal, Inc.
PO Box 5312
Santa Monica, CA 90409
(800) 800-0405

Health Concerns
2415 Mariner Sq. Drive, #3
Alameda, CA 94501
(800) 233-9355

Priesont and Associates
(Southern California only)
(310) 379-0271

Granular extracts:
Sun Ten Formulas
Brion Corporation
9250 Jeronimo Road
Irvine, CA 92718
(800) 333-4372

Qualiherb
13340 E. Firestone Bld.
Suite N
Santa Fe Springs, CA 90670
(800) 533-5907

Kanpo Formulas
Kanpo
PO Box 60279
Sacramento, CA 95860
(916) 487-9044

Mintang Formulas
Tashi Enterprises
429 Ashbury Ave.
El Cerrito, CA 94530
(415) 524-7913

Health Concerns
Health Concerns
2415 Mariner Sq. Drive, # 3
Alameda, CA 94501
(800) 233-9355

K'an Herb Company
Jade Pharmacy
K'an Herb Company
2425 Porter Street
Soquel, CA 95073
(408) 462-9915

Crane Enterprises
45 Samoset Ave, RFD #1
Plymouth, MA 02360
(800) 227-4118

Health Concerns
2415 Mariner Square Drive,
Suite 3
Alameda, CA 94501
(800) 233-9355

Chinese herbal
patent medicines:
K'an Herb Company
2425 Porter Street
Soquel, CA 95073
(408) 462-9915

Mayway Trading Company
780 Broadway
San Francisco, CA 92133
(415) 788-3646

Southwest Acupunc.College
712 W. San Mateo
Santa Fe, NM 87501
(505) 988-3538